Specific Medication and Specific Medicines

John Milton Scudder

257

SPECIFIC MEDICATION

AND

SPECIFIC MEDICINES.

REVISED,

WITH AN APPENDIX CONTAINING THE ARTICLES PUBLISHED
ON THE SUBJECT SINCE THE FIRST EDITION.

AND A

REPORT OF CASES ILLUSTRATING SPECIFIC MEDICATION.

BY

JOHN M. SCUDDER, M. D.,

PROFESSOR OF THE PRINCIPLES AND PRACTICE OF MEDICINE IN THE ECLECTIC
MEDICAL INSTITUTE; AUTHOR OF "THE PRINCIPLES OF MEDICINE,"
"THE ECLECTIC PRACTICE OF MEDICINE," "THE ECLECTIC
MATERIA MEDICA AND THERAPEUTICS," "A PRACTICAL
TREATISE ON THE DISEASES OF WOMEN," ETC.

FOURTH EDITION.

CINCINNATI:
WILSTACH, BALDWIN & CO., PRINTERS.
1873.

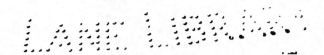

PREFACE.

For some hundred years or more, there has been a pretty uniform agreement in the statement, so frequently repeated— " there are no specifics in medicine." To have a good reputation for professional acquirements and standing, this was a fundamental article of belief. Whatever might be the certainty in Anatomy, Physiology, Chemistry, and the arts of the Obstetrician and Surgeon, it was essential to believe that the practice of medicine was a great uncertainty.

That it was a great uncertainty, as commonly followed, we are well assured. The records of disease, the mortality tables, and the resultant lesions from the mal-administration of medicines, abundantly testify to this.

This stands confessed in the writings of the most prominent men in the medical profession to-day, who unite in deprecating the use of the older treatment of disease, and the greater safety of the *expectant* plan—which is really diet and rest.

Must we give up medicine entirely? Are there no agencies opposed to processes of disease, that we can employ with certainty? These are the questions of the day, and in answering them, we will decide either for no medicine, or for specific medication.

To determine which of these shall be chosen, the reader will have to refer to his own experience of the action of medicines, and be guided by it. All will admit the uncertainty of medicine, as now used, but no one will be willing to confess that he really knows nothing in therapeutics. I think it will be safe to assert that every practitioner will have the knowl-edge of some antagonism of medicine to disease, that is clear, definite and uniform. If he has but one such, it is positive proof there are others, and the evidence that direct or specific medication is a possibility.

Specific medication requires specific diagnosis. We do not propose to teach that single remedies are opposed to diseases according to our present nosology. These consist of an asso-ciation of functional and structural lesions, varying in degree and combination at different times, very rarely the same in any two cases. To prescribe remedies rationally, we are required to analyze the disease and separate it into its component ele-ments, and for these we select the appropriate remedy.

The writer has had a sufficiently extended experience in the treatment of disease, to say that he knows absolutely that remedies have this direct antagonistic action to disease, and in many instances he is able to define it so that the reader can readily determine its truth. Still the field of investigation is a broad one, it has been but little cultivated, and there are few careful observers, so that much of the work remains for future investigation.

The tendency of medicine in all schools, however, is in the one direction. The giving up of the old uncertainty is the first step, then follows the careful study of individual reme-dies, and their use to accomplish certain well defined objects. One need not be a prophet to forecast the future in this respect. The medicine of the future will very certainly be *direct*, or as we have chosen to term it, "Specific Medication."

The object of the author has been to make the subject as plain as possible, and not to obscure it with useless verbiage. The first intention was to tell only what he knew—then this small volume would have been but a pamphlet. But on further consideration it was deemed best, to point out the lines of investigation with the larger number of our indigenous medicines, that they might be thoroughly tested.

No apology is offered for its shortcomings. It has been compiled in considerable part, from monthly articles in the Eclectic Medical Journal, and is presented to the profession as a guide in part, but especially as an incentive to the re-study of the Materia Medica.

PREFACE TO FOURTH EDITION.

In presenting the profession a revised edition of this little work, the author wishes to return his thanks for the kindness with which it has been received, and the attention that has been given the subject. No one knows better the prejudices that are arrayed against any new doctrine in medicine, and how closely many physicians wrap themselves in the mantle of the "fathers," lest anything new should reach them. Yet we have had a fair hearing, and the facts presented have been very thoroughly tested, and so far as the results have been learned, the experience is in favor of "Specific Medication."

The author regrets that he has not been able to do more in this direction, and especially that he has not the results of the thousands of experiments that have been made by others in the past two years. Every one has been studying Specific Medication for himself, and as the majority are workers, not writers, we have but a meager report of what has been done—yet this is most encouraging.

We don't propose, however, to give it up at this stage. We take up the labor of years, proposing to carry it on so long as life and health are spared, and with the aid that others will give, we hope to make the next edition meet the wishes of all the friends of a rational practice of medicine.

AVONDALE, April, 1873.

SPECIFIC MEDICATION

AND

SPECIFIC MEDICINES.

THE THEORY OF SPECIFIC MEDICATION.

I take it for granted that the reader will concede that all agents employed as medicines act either upon function or structure, and that this action to be curative must be opposed to the processes of disease. This proposition seems so plain that it requires no presentation of facts in proof, yet it is well to give it careful consideration, and arrange such facts as may have come under the reader's observation in its support.

If the action of a remedy is to oppose a process of disease, evidently its selection will depend—first, upon a correct knowledge of the disease, and second, upon a correct knowledge of this opposition of remedies to it.

It is a law of the universe, "that like causes always produce like effects," or to reverse it, "that like effects always flow from like causes." Therefore, if we can determine the opposition of a remedy to a process of disease in any given case, we have determined it in all like cases. And, to make use of this knowledge subsequently it is only necessary that we be able to determine the *exact* condition of disease, when we very certainly expect to obtain the same curative (opposing) action from the remedy.

In describing this action to another, it is necessary—first, that we so observe and group the signs and symptoms of disease, that he may get the exact idea of the pathological condition to be opposed. The skill required is in diagnosis, and necessitates a very thorough re-study of pathology, ignoring to a great extent, our present nosology. To facilitate this study, the author has published a work—" The Principles of Medicine "—which embodies his views, and will serve as a basis for specific or direct medication. Much that might be deemed necessary in this monograph, will there be found in its proper connection, and we have not deemed it desirable to separate it and reproduce it here.

Many persons are in error in regard to *our* use of the term *specific*. They think of a *specific medicine*, as one that will cure all cases of a certain disease, according to our present nosology, as pneumonitis, dysentery, diarrhœa, albuminuria, phthisis, etc. ; and a person looking at the subject in this light, and guided by his experience in the use of remedies, would at once say there are no specifics.

We use the term *specific* with relation to definite pathological conditions, and propose to say, that certain well determined deviations from the healthy state, will always be corrected by certain specific medicines.

A disease, according to our present nosology, may be formed of one, or of a half-dozen or more distinct pathological changes, bearing a determinate relation to one another. We do not propose to reach all of these by one remedy, except in those cases in which one lesion is primary, and the others result from it. But on the contrary, we propose a remedy for each pathological feature, using the remedy for that first which is first in the chain of morbid action, and that second which stands second, and so on.

As an example, we analyze a case of fever, and find it to consist of a lesion of the circulation, a lesion of innervation, a lesion of secretion, a lesion of the blood, and a lesion of nutrition; each of these is regarded as a distinct element of the disease, but in the order named,—the one depending upon the other to a certain extent. A remedy that will rectify the lesion of circulation, will sometimes be sufficient to arrest the entire chain of morbid phenomena—as we notice in the simple fevers. Or a remedy that will correct the lesion of the blood— this being primary and the cause of the various morbid processes,—will be a *specific* for all, as when quinine arrests an intermittent or remittent fever.

But in the severer types of disease, we find it necessary to use a remedy or remedies for each pathological feature. Thus, we employ one to correct the lesion of circulation, one to correct the lesion of innervation, special remedies to increase secretion, to correct the lesion of the blood, etc. Instead of one remedy to arrest the disease, according to the ordinary use of the term specific, we employ a number of different agents, which are none the less specific, for they meet distinct features of the diseased action.

To employ remedies in this way, it is requisite that we analyze the disease according to what we know of pathology, determining definitely the elements that go to form it, and their relation to one another.

And secondly, that we know the direct influence of remedies upon the human body, both in health and disease; that we use them singly or in simple combinations; that we do one thing at a time: that first which is first, that second which holds the second place, and so on.

If one expects to obtain the advantages of *specific* medication, he must not associate it with *indirect* medication. The direct sedatives, with free podophyllin catharsis — veratrum in pneumonia, with nauseants, blisters, etc., are incompatible. Success comes from one or the other alone. If I use *direct* medication I use it alone, and if I use *indirect* medication I use it alone. If we propose to treat a case of croup with Aconite, we do not use nauseants; if we propose to cure a case of cholera infantum with Ipecac and Nux Vomica, we do not want astringents.

But we go further into the analysis of diseased

action as expressed by symptoms, than many suppose. The success of direct medication comes from the definiteness of diagnosis—determining the *exact* condition of a function or part.

To illustrate, it is not sufficient in selecting a sedative to know that the pulse is frequent, using alike Veratrum, Aconite, Digitalis, Gelseminum, or Lobelia. Frequency is but one element of the lesion : and we have to determine in addition the strength or weakness of the circulation, the degree of obstruction of the capillary circulation, and the condition of the nervous system that controls this function. Thus, where there is strength with frequency we employ Veratrum ; feebleness with frequency, Aconite ; excitation of the nervous system with strength and frequency, Gelseminum ; atony of the nervous system and tendency to stasis of blood, Aconite and Belladonna ; feeble impulse from the heart, without capillary obstruction, Digitalis, etc.

It is not sufficient to know that the tongue is coated, indicating an impairment or arrest of digestion. We make this secretion give us the history of blood lesions, as well as of gastric and intestinal derangements. We learn that *pallid* mucous membranes with white coat demand alkalies ; that *deep red* mucous membranes and brown coat call for acids ; that a dirty-white, pasty coat requires the alkaline sulphites, etc. It is not necessary to continue this illustration further, for the reader will see by the above that the *specific medication* requires spe-

cific diagnosis, and that it will be successful just in proportion as we become skilled in this.

It is true that almost any one can use Veratrum and Aconite successfully, for the conditions are so prominent that they can not be mistaken; or any one may successfully prescribe Aconite in sporadic dysentery from cold; Ipecac in the diarrhœa of children; Collinsonia or Hamamelis for hemorrhoids; Collinsonia for ministers' sore throat; Cactus for heart disease; Pulsatilla for nervousness; Staphysagria for prostatorrhœa; Eryngium Aquaticum for cystic or urethral irritation; Apocynum Canabinum for dropsy, etc., etc. These remedies have an extra value attached to them, because the conditions indicating them are so easily determined.

Yet the reader will learn with surprise that ten years since, with but one exception, not one of these agents were used for the purpose named. In 1860, 10 lbs. of the crude root of Collinsonia supplied the market for a year; now one house gets in 10,000 lbs. for the year's supply.

SPECIFIC DIAGNOSIS.

We have already insisted upon the necessity of specific diagnosis if we are to expect definite curative action from medicines. This is a very important element of specific or direct medication that many physicians do not seem to understand. When we speak of specific medication they get the idea of an absolute cure for disease according to our present nosology, and say there is no such thing as a specific medicine. They expect to guess at the name of a disease, and find a remedy that will fit their guess-work. To suit such, a medicine must be like a blunderbuss, scattering its shot all over the field, giving a probability that some will reach the mark.

Direct medication, on the contrary, requires *specific diagnosis*. We must know exactly what the departure from health is, and knowing this we may select a remedy which will correct it. As was remarked before, the physician must have first a thorough knowledge of *healthy* life, and be able to recognize it, or any departure from it. Thus Anatomy and Physiology are the true basis of direct medication, for if we do not know the healthy structure and function, it is not possible that we can *know* the diseased structure and function.

We have a very simple rule for measuring the departure from health, and it is easily applied. It is in one of three directions—*excess, defect,* or *perversion*—above, below, or from. If we can measure disease in this way, the desired remedial action is at once suggested—if in excess it is to be diminished, if defective it is to be increased, if perverted it is to be brought back to the normal standard. In a majority of acute diseases, we will find these departures so clearly marked that the diagnosis and treatment are very easy.

But as there are many elements that go to make healthy life in man, so there are many that go to make the sum of disease. These will be found in varying combination, yet in most cases there are certain prominent lesions which may be regarded as standing first in the chain of morbid phenomena and upon which the others rest. If we can find remedies which will reach and correct these, the disease is at an end, and the natural restorative power of the body soon gives health.

The most simple form of specific medication is where a single remedy is sufficient to arrest the process of disease. As when we prescribe Collinsonia for ministers' sore throat, Drosera for the cough of measles, Belladonna for congestive headache, Macrotys for muscular pains, Hamamelis for hemorrhoids, Phytolacca for mammary irritation, Cactus for functional heart disease, Staphysagria for prostatorrhœa, etc. This use of remedies gives great satisfaction in the treatment of many diseases, and we are led to wish that the practice of medicine could be resolved into the giving of such specifics.

Not quite so simple, but yet very plain is the second form of direct medication, illustrated by the following examples. A heavily loaded tongue at base, with a bad taste in the mouth and fullness in the epigastric region, demanding an emetic. A uniformly yellowish coated tongue from base to tip, relieved by Podophyllin or Leptandrin. A pallid tongue, coated white, calling for a salt of soda. A pallid large tongue, with a moist pasty coat, demanding the alkaline sulphites, say sulphite of soda. The deep red tongue and mucous membranes with brownish coatings, demanding the use of acids, say muriatic acid.

Quite as plain, but not so easily and directly reached by medicine, is the need of a good condition of the intestinal canal for digestion and blood making, and associated with it the recognition of the need of certain restoratives that may be necessary to normal nutrition and functional activity. These are essentials in the treatment of every form of disease. In acute cases, it is required first to rid our patient of functional disease before we can fully establish digestion and nutrition, but in chronic disease it will many times stand first, and must always be associated with treatment for local lesions.

The complement of this is, treatment to increase the removal of old and worn-out tissues, and thus relieve the solids and fluids of material that must necessarily depress functional activity. Probably we have as little positive knowledge of remedies that increase retrograde metamorphosis, as of any other class, still they are being studied, and in time we will be enabled to use them directly. Remedies that increase excretion are in common use, and form a very important part of our practice. From the earliest periods of medicine, the fact that disease is destructive has been recognized. Destruction of the material of our bodies, necessarily leaves the debris either in solids or fluids, and experience has shown that it can not remain in the body with safety. Hence the common use of those agents

that stimulate excretion from skin, kidneys and
bowels.

But there has been a failure to appreciate the
true nature of these processes, and from this has
flowed a very great deal of bad practice. These
processes are strictly vital processes, carried on by
delicate organisms under the control of the nervous
system. As they are the basis of life, we may well
suppose that nature has guarded them on all sides,
and that they are the true centre of life. The doctor of the olden time has looked upon them as
mechanisms to be powerfully influenced by remedies. He powerfully excites the stomach and intestinal canal as a means of derivation, and works
upon the skin and kidneys as if secretion from them
were a purely physical process. Thousands of lives
have been and are being destroyed in this way.
Any one who will take up Huxley's Physiology,
and read the clear and simple description of this
apparatus for digestion and waste, upon which our
lives rest, can not but be satisfied that the common
practice of medicine is a very great wrong. A man
lives, because he has the power of renewing his life
day by day. Take away this power and he will die
in a brief time; take it away in part, and you have
lessened his power to that extent; take it away for
an hour, for a day, or for a week, and his power to
live is weakened to that extent.

When we regard these processes as strictly vital
processes, in highly developed organs, under the
control of a most delicately adjusted nervous system,

we will be in a position to use remedies to aid vital action. Studying the condition of the stomach and intestinal canal in this light, we will see how a direct stimulant, or tonic, an alkali, an acid, a remedy that will relieve nervous irritation, or one that will give increased innervation, will in different cases be an aid to digestion. Looking farther, we will see the necessity, in one case of histogenetic food, in another of calorifacient, in one of iron, in another of phosphorus, etc. It is just as much *specific medication* to be able to select the proper food for the sick as it is the proper medicine.

One or two examples of this may not be out of place. The past winter I was called in consultation, in a case of continued fever in the third week. The treatment, so far as medicine was concerned, had been very judicious, but the food had been starchy, and for a week the patient had been able to take very little. He was failing fast, and stimulants and tonics were used without advantage. The most striking features of the disease to me were: the feebleness of the heart's action, the want of respiratory power, and the evidences of a general failure of muscular power—in all other respects the patient was in good condition. I advised enemata of beef-essence, and its internal administration in small quantities frequently repeated, and a suspension of all medicine. The effect was marked in twenty-four hours, and the patient speedily recovered. In the early part of my practice I had occasion to call Dr. William Judkins in consultation, in the case of a lady who had incipient phthisis developed from menstrual irregularity. She was very feeble, and I had been giving her freely of the bitter tonics, stimulants and animal food. The old Quaker remarked, if thee will stop the medicine and stimulants, and give her fatty matter she will recover—and the result justified the old doctor's skill in diagnosis. I have had to take this advice twice in the past eighteen months, from other parties, when I should have recognized it myself; in both it was the one thing necessary to success.

With regard to excretion, we must be thoroughly impressed with the fact that it is *wholly* a vital process, and not a process of straining. When we come to understand that a secreting organ is continually growing secreting cells, and that these withdraw from the blood the worn-out materials of our bodies, we will be in a position to use remedies with better success. Evidently it is possible to so over-stimulate or over-work an excretory organ, that this function of cell-production will be very much diminished or altogether arrested. Just in this proportion must secretion be impaired or wholly arrested. The best remedies to increase secretion are those that act mildly and stimulate vital function.

Thus far direct medication is very plain sailing. All can succeed with it, yet successes will be in proportion to the physician's acuteness of observation, and to some extent upon his knowledge of remedies. But beyond this we have a field that requires a very thorough knowledge of vital processes, accurate observation, and an extended knowledge of remedies. We study not so much the grosser manifestations of disease, but the more delicate shadings and combinations, and our therapeutics requires that we have a most intimate knowledge of the influence of remedies upon the human body. In this field of study the physician will find a beauty and certainty in the practice of medicine that will give zest to investigation, and as it is pursued he will find greater and greater success.

DIFFERENCE FROM HOMŒOPATHY.

The question has been asked, "In what does your theory of specific medication differ from Homœopathy?" The question is a pertinent one, and I will endeavor to answer it briefly.

The law, *similia similibus*, upon which the Homœopathic practice is based, is defined in two ways. One contends that the drug, used for cure, "produces the essential morbid condition" when proven in health. The other, "that it produces similar symptoms," but not the exact pathological condition.

The truth in this law of *similia similibus*, is, that certain agents, called medicines, act on particular organs, parts, and functions of the human body in a uniform manner. They act equally on the organ, part, or function, in health and disease; and thus acting in health, they produce such change in the phenomena of life as to render the action sensible

to the person—symptoms.   If an agent directly and
uniformly produces an influence upon a particular
part, it is more likely to be used as a remedy in disease of that part than another which does not influence the part at all.

Remedies are, therefore, those agents which
directly and uniformly influence an organ, part, or
function.   The question then comes up, are they
remedies because " they will produce a similar state
of disease," or because they are opposed to diseased
action ?

The Homœopaths will not admit any explanation
of their law of *similia*.   The remedy is a remedy
because it will produce the exact diseased condition,
or at least the exact symptoms of such condition.

I contend that a drug is a specific remedy: first,
because it influences uniformly and directly the
part or function diseased; and second, because it
opposes such diseased action.   I would, therefore,
write the law of cure, *contraria contrariis opponenda*,
instead of *similia similibus*.

I find a late authority in Homœopathy agrees
with me in this.   Dr. v. Grauvogl, in his " Lehr-
buch Der Homœopathy," says:—" The conception
of a specific reme ly expresses the mutual relation
existing between it and parts of the organism,
which has to be ascertained empirically by physiological provings of drugs.   For some part of the
organism is in a relation of immunity, for other
parts of attraction, for others again one of repulsion,
and always *vice versa*.   For instance, there is a spe-

cific form of fever and ague which, for these very reasons, is cured by Quinine, a dose or quantity of Quinine being given which corresponds to the intensity of the attack."

Again with reference to the dose of medicines: "All we have to do is to determine, independently of all subjective persuasions and incomprehensibilities, what quantity of a substance is necessary in order to produce in any morbidly affected part of the organism a chemical or physical counter-movement of equal intensity, and in an opposite direction to the movement originated by the morbific cause, with a view of arresting, or at least, retarding this latter, and finally discontinuing it altogether by repeating the dose.   *   *   *   The problem is simply to determine what remedial movement quantities will antagonize as their equivalent the movements that had been excited by the morbific agent; for the measure of the force is the effect, nothing else. To solve this problem we have the natural law according to which quantity contains the measure of the movement and counter-movement; consequently for therapeutic purposes, the correct dose consists in a quantity of force of the indicated quality which is equal to the quantity of force of the morbific agent, and in its movements runs in a contrary direction to the quality of the latter."

In ordinary practice, whether it be Old School or Eclectic, there is no *principle* or *law* of cure. Remedies are not given because they are opposed to or agree with diseased action, but simply because they have been previously used with reputed good success. It is, in fact, pure empiricism. The old dogma of phlogosis and antiphlogistics, and the new doctrine of impaired vitality and restorative medication, guides the empirical use of remedies in the one or other direction.

THE ADMINISTRATION OF MEDICINES.

We may lay it down as an *axiom*, from which it is never safe to depart, that—*No medicine should be given, unless the pathological condition and the indications for its use are clearly defined.* It is much better to employ a *placebo*, than run the risk of doing harm by medication.

Good nursing is an essential element in the successful practice of medicine, and always requires direction by the physician; keeping the stomach in good condition for the reception of food and medicine, is of first importance, and requires attention. Following this is the selection of proper food, its preparation, and the time for its administration. These alone very well repay the careful attention and thought of the physician, even if he can not see an indication for the employment of remedies.

When we recollect that the cause of disease is always depressing, and a source of constant renewal, we will see that the removal of the cause from the patient or the patient from the cause, or the antagonism of remedies to remove the cause, is a proper field for our efforts. If we can see clearly that the condition of disease is one of depression—that in proportion as a man is sick, his vitality is lessened, such means as will increase the power to live, or the resistance of the body to death, will be suggested.

As we have stated before, we make an analysis of the disease and divide it into its component parts, before making a prescription of medicine. There are certain *basic* functions or conditions upon which all others rest, and which are essential to life. These demand our first consideration. Thus the *circulation of the blood*, the *temperature*, the *condition of the nervous system, waste, excretion*, the *condition of the blood, blood-making* and *nutrition*, are examined separately. Determining the lesion of these, we prescribe such remedy as antagonizes it, and brings the function toward the healthy standard. Some one of them will stand first in the series of pathological changes, and will serve as a basis for others, and this will receive first attention. Thus we prescribe at the other lesions, in the order in which they seem to be arranged.

As a rule, *it is best to do one thing at a time.* We prescribe first for that lesion which *is* first in the chain of morbid action. Then maintaining the influence obtained by a continuation of the remedy, we do that second which is second, and that third which is third, and so on.

In the cure of disease *time* is an important element, and it is never best to be in a hurry. Here,

3

the old proverb "haste makes waste," is a very true one. As a rule, the severer the disease, the slower its development; the slower the departure from health the greater the impairment of function and structure, and necessarily the slower its restoration.

The manifestations of life in man are from a highly developed organism, the perfection of which is a work of time. Every manifestation of life necessitates a continued renewal of structure, requiring an expenditure of that force we know as vital. Therefore, when the manifestations of life are abnormal (disease), we must necessarily allow time for the development of the organism, increased because the vital force is impaired.

As a rule, *it is best to change the manifestations of diseased life slowly*, giving sufficient time for the organism to adapt itself to the change, and gain increased strength as it returns to the condition of health. It will never do to suppress a process of disease at the risk of suppressing the organism upon which natural function depends.

As a rule, *it is best to effect these changes insensibly, or without shock to an organ or to the entire body.* In this, as in all other things, it is the slow but continued application of an opposing force, that accomplishes the greatest results. Many thousands of sick have been hurried to their graves by the sudden and forcible efforts of the physician to remove disease. This is one of the most prominent

errors of the old practice, and will require considerable effort to avoid.

As a rule, *it is best to employ remedies singly, or in
simple combination of remedies acting in the same way.*
The reasons for this rule are obvious. It prevents
random or scattering prescriptions. We either
know a *single* remedy that will accomplish the object, or we know nothing and have no right to
make a prescription. There can not be anything in
a combination that is not in the individual articles
composing it, and in some one of them *par excellence :*
this is the remedy to use. In direct medication we
want no modifying influences ; we want the plain
and constant action of a simple remedy.

THE FORM OF MEDICINE.

The common action of many medicines obtained
in the old practice is the poisonous action. The
agent is given in such large doses and is so *nauseous*,
that the human body in self-preservation is forced
to act upon and expel it. Thus, an emetic forces
the stomach to an act of expulsion, and we have
emesis ; a cathartic influences the intestinal canal
in like manner and we have catharsis ; and so with
diaphoretics and diuretics. A different class, which
may be represented by mercury, antimony, and
arsenic, obtain entrance to the blood, and depressing
this, they depress every manifestation of life until
they are finally slowly removed.

If we desire to obtain these grave influences of

medicine, the form is not particular, neither is the size of the dose—if the patient can stand it. But if we desire that slow, insensible, but direct action that I have spoken of, we want our remedies in such form that they will be kindly received and have a kindly action upon the organism.

We have also to take into consideration the preservation of the article, uniformity of action, pleasantness to the sick, portability, and ease of prescription. These hold a secondary place, yet are very important.

A class of remedies may be regarded as chemicals, and these we desire in greatest purity, and only purchase such as bear the names of the best manufacturers. Such are Quinia, Morphia, Sulphite of Soda, Phosphate of Soda, the Bromides, etc.

The largest class is obtained from the vegetable world, and are products of nature's laboratory. These we wish unchanged by art, as nature has prepared them, simply reducing the bulk, and using a vehicle to preserve them.

Very certainly the best menstruum for all vegetable remedies is alcohol and water in varying proportion. There is no vegetable product that does not yield its medicinal properties to these, in a very concentrated form, the alcohol being in sufficient proportion for preservation. Not only so, but with modern apparatus for percolation, the fluid may easily represent the strength of ounce for ounce, giving sufficient concentration to make it portable.

The tincture thus prepared is miscible with water,

which is undoubtedly the best vehicle for the introduction of a remedy into the blood. In using a
hypodermic injection, we employ water as a vehicle
for the medicine, and not simple syrup, syrup of
lemon or ginger, an extract of quassia or other
nasty substance, and so in introducing remedies
into the circulation, through the stomach, we will
find water decidedly the best vehicle.

Remedies in *pura naturalibus* are not offensive, it
is the covering them up, and mixing them that
makes them unpleasant. Doctors' potions are proverbially nasty, and the public mind has been cultivated to believe that a mixture in a bottle must be
an offence to smell, taste and stomach. The
thoughts of such medicines are enough to make
some sick.

My prescriptions are uniformly made with water
as a vehicle, the tincture being added to it in such
proportion that the dose will be a teaspoonful. If
the tinctures are carried in the pocket case, we add
them to a glass of water in proper proportion, and
renew the medicine at each visit that it may be
fresh.

In the treatment of diseases of children this extemporaneous dispensing is especially desirable.
Children are naturally adverse to anything unpleasant, and one ordinary drugging is sufficient to
" put them against medicine." It is very unpleasant
to be required to force medicine upon a child against
its wishes, still more to throw it down, hold it for-
cibly, and grasping its nose make it swallow the

mixture. No wonder parents turn from such practice to Homœopathy.

It has been my practice to have the little patient
see all the operations of preparing the medicine.
It sees the pocket case, inspects the bottles, and is
convinced that everything is clean and there is
nothing objectionable. The glass of water is placed
before it, and the few drops of medicine added, and
to the request, " My dear, taste this and see if the
medicine is not good," it offers no objection, is satisfied, and you have obtained the little patient's
confidence, and will never lose it until you abuse it.

THE DOSE OF MEDICINE.

As a rule, *the dose of medicine should be the smallest
quantity that will produce the desired result.* The
proper dose, or that which gives the best result, is
very much smaller than one who has been used to
the large doses of indirect medicine would suppose
possible. Yet it is not infinitesimal, as our Homœopathic friends would have us believe. It is difficult
to state what the dose should be as yet, but I believe those named in connection with the remedies
are the *maximum.*

A few examples may serve to illustrate this. In
the olden time we thought the dose of a strong
tincture of Macrotys was from half to one teaspoonful, repeated every two or three hours, until " the
head felt like bursting." I now find the remedy
much more certain in the proportion of 3j. of the

tincture to water ℥iv. a teaspoonful every two hours. The common directions for using Veratrum (Norwood's Tincture) were to commence with a dose of three drops every three hours, increasing one drop each dose, until its full effect was produced. Now the dose is always less than one drop. Aconite was formerly given in doses of drops, now in fractions of drops.

The dose will vary in different cases, and with different practitioners. If it falls below the gross or poisonous action of the drug, it will have specific influence, and the diagnosis being right, will accomplish the object of the prescriber. I am satisfied that the size of the dose does not make such difference as has been thought, and that the essential element of success is to get the *right* remedy.

THE PREPARATION OF REMEDIES.

The majority of physicians will prepare but few remedies themselves, yet it is just as essential that they know how they should be prepared, as if they made them all. With an intelligent understanding of the simpler processes of pharmacy, he will have a much better knowledge of the physical properties of medicines, and be enabled to judge somewhat of their purity and efficiency when purchasing.

The general drug trade has been a miserable fraud upon the profession. Whether selling crude or manufactured articles, the chances were ten to one that they were adulterated, and not what they were represented, (Morphia, Quinia, and some of the common chemicals, have been exceptions.)

So far has this sophistication been carried that all certainty in medicine, even in gross drugging for indirect effect, has been lost. Solid or fluid extracts are found of all degrees of strength, from the highest named in the pharmacopœia to nothing. In many cases they are prepared from old and worthless crude material, that has partly or wholly lost its medicinal properties, yet it is sold in the same packages and at the same prices, as if good.

There is but one safe plan for the physician in procuring remedies, and that is by personal experiment to satisfy himself that a *good* remedy can be readily prepared, and learn to know it when he sees it. Deal with houses that claim to prepare remedies from recent crude material, of full strength, without heat, and return every package that does not come up to the full standard of strength and excellence.

It is well to adopt a simple nomenclature for fluid medicines. Let them be called *tinctures*, as they are prepared with alcohol, and specify the strength ounce for ounce, of crude material to fluid preparation.

I insist that all vegetable remedies should be prepared from the *recent* crude material obtained at its proper season. In some cases the remedy does not materially deteriorate within the year, and may be kept in stock until the next season for gathering. But in all cases it is better if prepared at once after gathering, and in many the preparation should be from the *fresh* article before any dessication. The reasons are obvious—the medicinal properties are found in the juices of the plant, or stored in its cells, principally of the bark. In both cases drying removes the medicinal principle, to a greater or less extent. The medicinal principles of plants are to a considerable extent complex and unstable organic bodies, and time, with its constant processes of change and decay, changes, deteriorates, and finally destroys them.

STRENGTH OF FLUID REMEDIES. — As before re-marked, a remedy is desirable in proportion as it is easily carried and dispensed, (leaving out of the question its medicinal action), hence concentration becomes an important element of pharmacy. A skilled manufacturer who has the proper appliances, has no difficulty in removing all the medicinal prop-erties from vegetable products, so that one Troy ounce of crude material will be contained in one fluid-ounce of the tincture.

This may be accomplished by the simple process of percolation, in most cases. In some pharmacies this is supplemented by powerful pressure; in other cases, the hydraulic press being employed with ad vantage. In other establishments, the new process of percolation under atmospheric pressure, has been adopted with great advantage. Either of these methods if carefully and honestly conducted will give reliable and uniform remedies. If we can make up our minds that it is quality, rather than quantity, that we should look after, slight variations

of strength will make but little difference. I do
not wish to be understood, however, as admitting that there can be any great variation of
medicinal strength, if recent crude material is used,
and the product represents ounce for ounce, and
the pharmaceutical processes have been skillfully
conducted.

PHYSICAL PROPERTIES OF FLUID REMEDIES.—The
fluid preparations should possess the exact physical
properties (intensified), as regards odor and taste,
of the fresh crude material. It will have the color
of the chlorophyll of the article, but should be
clear and transparent, and give no sediment, or
muddiness when shaken. These may seem like
minor matters, yet we will find it profitable to give
them attention. Skilled pharmacy gives fine looking remedies, and they are likely to be good. Un-
skilled pharmacy gives dirty-looking preparations,
and they are likely to be inferior.

We may judge to a considerable extent of the
goodness of chemicals in the same way. If we find
our Sulphate of Quinia and Morphia presenting the
clear white silky or feathered crystals, we are satisfied that we have good remedies. But if it is dull,
discolored, crystals faint, broken, or amorphous, we
want none of it. So in the purchase of the Bromides, Iodides, Salts of Potash and Soda, Iron, etc.,
we expect to find the highest physical qualities,
associated with purity and efficiency. If a salt is
discolored, or in any wise deficient in its appearance, we want none of it.

OFFICE PHARMACY.

There are good reasons why every physician should have such knowledge of pharmacy, that he can perform or direct all the simpler operations for preparing medicines. Without this knowledge, his education is deficient, in that he has not that knowledge of his *tools* which is so essential to good work. He is in a condition to be imposed upon by imperfect and worthless remedies, and must surely lose confidence in medicine, except given in large doses, for its gross effects.

In country practice, a knowledge and practice of office pharmacy is an important element of success. The preparation of a remedy gives an interest in it that leads to thorough study and careful use. We learn what a good preparation is, and its advantages over the common stock in the drug trade, and we will afterward use more care in making our purchases. It economizes time, saves money, and cultivates habits of thrift, all of which are deficient in the medical profession.

It is not only an excellent school for the physician himself, but is also an admirable school for the student. It is a study of the Materia Medica, that gives a practical knowledge of remedies, and impresses the mind through the organs of sense, leaving lasting impressions.

I do not wish to be understood as advising the preparation of *all* medicines; or keeping the office dirty and unsightly with the refuse of roots, barks, and herbs. This is the opposite of what we desire; skill is associated with neatness and cleanliness. I know some pharmacists that are so slovenly and dirty in person and surroundings, that I should not like to take their medicines. (The only one who ever offered an objection to office pharmacy, had these faults in excess.)

A half dozen neat tin percolators of the capacity of two to ten pounds, hung in a closet or cupboard, with a large mortar, comprises the apparatus. The alcohol is kept in stock, and the crude material is procured at proper seasons and used fresh, or in some cases is ordered of the wholesale druggist when obtaining other medicines.

The process of percolation is a very simple one. The crude material requires to be as finely comminuted and as closely packed in the percolator as possible. It is then covered with alcohol, and allowed to stand for forty-eight hours, when the tincture is drawn off. Filter it through paper, and you have a fine looking remedy, that will give satisfaction whenever used.

In office pharmacy I have advised the strength to be ℥viij. of the crude material to the pint of alcohol, because it is more easily manipulated by one who is not expert. All the formula in this work are of this strength, for every remedy named may be prepared in the office.

The physician in the country will probably prepare only those remedies that are indigenous, and at the proper season the year's supply. It is not very difficult to find some one to gather the crude material, and the preparation comes at that season when there is least to do.

CLASSIFICATION OF REMEDIES.

I have been in doubt in regard to the best plan of arranging the remedies in this study. Evidently the old classification will not serve our purpose, for it deals with indirect action; and the influence of remedies in poisonous doses. We have not advanced far enough to make a new classification; at least, to make one that would facilitate our study. I have, therefore, concluded to take up the different articles in alphabetical order, and so far as possible make a brief review of our entire Materia Medica.

When a remedy has no especial value, it will be named so; and when it seems to have a specific action, not fully determined, this will be pointed out for future experiment. Self-deception is a very unprofitable pursuit, and great care will therefore be employed to insure accuracy, and no statement máde unless pretty thoroughly proven.

The best preparations, and the best process for office manufacture. will be given, also the form in which we deem it desirable to use them.

When we have thus given the Materia Medica a review, we will be better able to make a classification.

Some suggestions, however, as to the general indications for treatment, and use of remedies, may not be out of place, and will serve as a further illustration of our idea of specific medication.

In all acute, and most chronic diseases, our examination of the patient and our therapeutics will take this order: 1. With reference to the condition of the stomach and intestinal canal—bringing them to as nearly a normal condition as possible, that remedies may be kindly received and appropriated, and that sufficient food may be taken and digested. 2. With reference to the circulation of the blood, and the temperature—obtaining a normal circulation as regards frequency and freedom, and a temperature as near 98° as possible. 3. With reference to the presence of a *zymotic* poison, or other cause of disease—which may be neutralized, antagonized or removed. 4. With reference to the condition of the nervous system—giving good innervation. 5. With reference to the processes of waste and excretion—that the worn-out or enfeebled material may be broken down and speedily removed from the body. 6. With reference to blood-making and repair—that proper material be furnished for the building of tissue, and that the processes of nutrition are normally conducted.

These are general outlines for the study of disease, and the action of remedies in antagonizing it, and may aid in giving direction to our study, and enable each one to make a classification of remedies for himself. A brief consideration of each one, with examples of the application of remedies,

though it will be a repetition, may be of advantage
to the student.

1. The condition of the stomach is of first importance in the treatment of disease. It must be
in such condition that it will receive remedies
kindly, and permit their speedy absorption, in order
that they give us the desired results. Surely, it is
not difficult to see the necessity of this, if we take
no further view than to obtain the curative action of remedies. If the stomach does not receive
a remedy kindly, is irritated by it, we can not expect ready absorption, or the complete curative
action. If the stomach throws out its juices, which
digest or decompose a remedy, we can not expect
its curative action. If the stomach is secreting
mucus in large quantity, if it is in that condition in
which it is but a receptacle or retainer, then we can
not expect the ready absorption of remedies, and
will not get their curative action.

We are accustomed to specify two conditions of
the stomach, which may be tolerably easily determined by constant symptoms, and which should
always be corrected. These are :—

Irritation of the stomach, marked by a reddened
(bright) tongue, elongated and pointed, with sometimes reddened and erect papillæ. It is accompanied with unpleasant sensations of constriction,
and tenderness on pressure over the epigastrium.
There may be nausea, retching, or vomiting; and
in the severer cases, when prolonged, an irritation

of the sympathetic, and finally of the spinal and
cerebral nervous systems.

Its treatment takes precedence of everything
else, for until removed we can not expect the kindly
or definite action of remedies.

The remedies employed for its removal are:
minute doses of Aconite; small doses of Ipecac or
Lobelia; Hydrocyanic Acid, or better, a preparation of the bark of the Peach tree; Rhubarb;
Bismuth. These may be aided by the external use
of the cold pack, hot fomentations, or rubefacient
application, and sometimes an enema to remove the
torpor of the lower bowel. From twelve to forty-
eight hours, is usually the time required to effect it.

But, the reader may ask, why if remedies are
specific, name so many for the relief of so simple a
pathological condition as gastric irritation? The
question is pertinent, and we will endeavor to
answer it. Each of these remedies has a direct action in this condition, and each may be relied upon
as a remedy. We choose the remedy, however,
with reference to the association of diseased action,
and in some cases one will be found best, in others
another.

b. The *atonic* stomach, with increased secretion
of mucus, and sometimes with considerable accumulations. It is marked by the broad tongue,
heavily coated at its base, bad taste in the mouth,
and feeling of weight and heaviness in the epigastrium. The symptoms are distinct, and can not be
mistaken.

When the condition is pronounced, in severer forms of disease, there is no means which will reach it so directly and speedily as an emetic. It needs to be prompt and thorough in action, not producing debility or leaving the organ irritable. If not requiring this, we may accomplish the same object by the use of the Alkaline Sulphites, followed by Nux Vomica.

· We have many minor lesions that can not be classified under these, to which we will find single remedies specific. Thus in simple nausea and vomiting, without irritation, we prescribe Nux Vomica. In typhoid disease, with tumid mucous tissues, the Baptisia. Increased mucous secretion with irritability, Oxide of Zinc. Imperfect gastric secretion, Hydrastis. Increased mucous secretion with impaired functional activity, minute doses of Podophyllin, etc.*

2. We recognize the fact, *that just in proportion to the variation of the circulation and temperature from the normal standard is the severity and activity of disease.* The more frequent the pulse, and the higher the temperature, the more active a zymotic poison, the more rapid the progress of local or general disease, and the less able the body to protect itself, or expel the cause of disease. The rule here is absolute, and there is no variation from it.

In therapeutics we find—*that just in proportion as the circulation and temperature can be brought to, and*

*See Practice of Medicine, page 27.

4

maintained at the normal standard, just in that proportion are the processes of disease arrested, and vital processes re-established.

These facts must surely have been noticed by observers, and we can only wonder that they have never been clearly stated, and practiced upon.

If we take as an example a case of fever, we will find that remedies that will reduce the pulse to a normal frequency, giving freedom to the circulation, will reduce the temperature, and that just in proportion as this is accomplished, the febrile symptoms disappear, and the various vital functions are re-established. If we maintain the circulation and temperature at this point, the fever must certainly cease.

In acute inflammation, the rapidity of the local disease and destruction of tissue, is in the ratio of frequency of pulse and increase of temperature. Just in proportion as we get a normal circulation with reference to frequency and freedom, and diminished temperature, just in that proportion the inflammatory process is arrested.

In *asthenic* inflammation we find another element in the pathology of the disease—a want of vital power, either in the whole or in the part. This must be antagonized by appropriate remedies. In others there is a zymotic or animal poison, which must be antagonized, destroyed, or removed.

In chronic disease the law is just as absolute as in the acute. Given, any disease of function or structure, with a pulse maintained constantly above

100 beats per minute, and a temperature above 100°, and the patient must die. The disease, as a general rule, will run its course rapidly to a fatal termination just in proportion to the extent of this deviation.

Recovery from chronic disease never takes place until the circulation and temperature approximate a normal standard. In any given case, the probabilities of cure are as the possibility of bringing and maintaining the circulation and temperature at the standard of health. The first evidences of amendment are announced by a diminution of frequency of pulse and a better circulation of blood, and by an equal temperature of the body, approximating 98°. These seem like dogmatic statements, and many will be inclined to dispute them, because opposed or not named by the common authorities on medicine, but it only requires observation without prejudice to prove each position.

We may claim then, that remedies influencing the circulation and temperature, toward the normal standard, are the most important of the Materia Medica.

In very many cases the lesion of the circulation has basic lesion, upon which others arise and are continued. When this is the case, the remedy that restores normal circulation removes all the diseased phenomena which rest upon it. Thus we will find lesions of secretion and excretion, lesions of innervation, of waste and nutrition, as well as the influence of zymotic causes, are in proportion to the rapidity of the circulation. Conversely, as the pulse comes down to the normal standard, and the blood circulates freely, just in that proportion we have a restoration of the secretions and excretions, better innervation, better digestion and blood-making, and a more active waste and repair.

Have we remedies that influence the circulation directly, giving a free and equal circulation, with diminution of frequency? Many of our readers will have asked this question before this, and answered it in the negative. Certain remedies will have been recommended to them as *special sedatives*, which they have used without the good results named and expected. How is this? It is a common failing with physicians to expect a desired result too soon, and endeavor to force it by large doses of medicine. This has been a common cause of failure in the use of Veratrum and Aconite. Others have purchased worthless medicines, which will readily account for the failure. Taking the article of Veratrum alone, and excepting Norwood's Tincture, nine-tenths that has been sold was wholly worthless as a medicine.

The theory with regard to the action of the class of special sedatives was erroneous. They were regarded as *depressants*, and diminished frequency of pulse was supposed to depend upon their depressing influence upon the heart. It was the common error of large doses and poisonous action. All of these remedies are active poisons in large doses, and death occurs in all by *cardiac syncope*. In the cases of Veratrum, Digitalis, Lobelia and Gelseminum, slowness of pulse is a prominent symptom of the poisonous action. In the case of Aconite, extreme frequency of pulse is produced by the poisonous action.

Iu medicinal doses (small), the influence of these remedies is that of a cardiac stimulant, and is undoubtedly through the sympathetic system of nerves, which controls the entire circulation of the blood—not only the action of the heart, but of all the blood-vessels to the most minute capillary. I contend that this influence removes obstruction to the free circulation of the blood, as well as gives power to heart and muscular fibre of arteries. As obstruction to free circulation is removed, it requires less effort to move the blood; as the power of moving the blood is increased there is less necessity of frequency of contraction upon the part of the heart.

As a rule, the time required to effect sedation will bear a distinct relation to the time required for the development of disease, and its average duration. Thus in an acute fever or inflammation from cold, the influence of the sedative may be promptly obtained, and the disease speedily arrested. In continued fever, the accession of the disease (in most cases), is slow in proportion to its duration and severity. Here there are grave lesions of function, possibly of structure, and we expect to obtain the influence of the sedative slowly.*

*See Principles of Medicine, pp. 219, 264. The Eclectic Practice of Medicine, page 94.

Whilst each of the remedies named as arterial
sedatives, Aconite, Veratrum, Digitalis, Gelseminum, Lobelia, exert a direct influence in this direction, they are not equally valuable in all cases.
The two first are pre-eminently the sedatives, their
action being more definite and stronger, and adapted
to a larger number of cases. The special adapta-
tion of each to special forms of diseased action is
named in the description of the remedy.

The temperature bears such a constant relation
to the frequency of pulse, and general condition of
the circulation, that a remedy which will correct
the one will also correct the other. Thus we find
in practice that just as we bring the pulse to the
normal standard by the use of an arterial sedative,
in the same degree we reduce the temperature.
This is the case in chronic as well as in acute disease. For instance, in a case of phthisis we find a
temperature of 101° associated with a pulse above
100 beats per minute ; if it is possible to bring the
pulse down to 80 the temperature comes down to
98° and a fraction. If this can be maintained we
find a cessation of tubercular deposit, and a repara-
tive process set up in the lungs.

We have some special means to influence the
temperature, outside of the remedies acting upon
the circulation. A full description of them would
be out of place here, but may be found in my Principles of Medicine, p. 40.

8. The field of therapeutics embraced in our third
proposition is very large, and will well repay careful

study. Whilst zymotic causes have been recognized in many of the severe acute diseases, but little has been done to determine their character, or the means to antidote them. Possibly the observations of Prof. Polli, with regard to the influence of the Alkaline Sulphites, was the first important step in this direction.

The presence of such blood poison is readily detected, and we have advanced so far in our knowledge of remedies, that in many cases we can select the antidote with much certainty. I do not wish to be understood as claiming that we have any remedies that will immediately unite with all of a zymotic poison in the blood, destroy it, and at once restore health. Such an influence could not reasonably be expected. But we have remedies which, introduced into the blood, will antagonize the zymotic poison, as it comes in contact with it, arresting its septic influence, or wholly destroying it. In some cases they act rapidly, in others slowly, but in all, if properly selected, with great certainty.

The principal remedies of this class are the Alkaline Sulphites, (Sulphite of Soda being in most common use) and the mineral acids. The rules for the selection of the one or the other of these are quite simple, and very definite:

In any given case presenting a pallid tongue, with white, or dirty-white, pasty coating, use the Alkaline Sulphites.

In any given case presenting a deep-red tongue with brownish coatings, or deep-red glossy tongue,

and dark sordes, use mineral acids.   In some cases
we employ Sulphurous Acid, but in the majority,
Muriatic Acid.

Of our indigenous Materia Medica we have but
one remedy that markedly possesses these properties, and it possesses it in high degree.   This remedy is the Baptisia Tinctoria, which may be used in
either of the cases named, but is especially valued
in the last.

The reader will bear in mind that the activity of
a zymotic poison is in exact proportion to the departure from normal function.   With a rapid pulse,
high temperature, and arrest of secretion, its development is rapid and its devitalizing influence
marked.   Or in the rare opposite case of congestive
intermittent and cholera, as the circulation is enfeebled, and the temperature lowered, its progress
is rapid.

Hence, in order to antagonize a zymotic process,
it is necessary, so far as possible, to obtain a normal
circulation and temperature.   This proposition can
not be too strongly insisted upon.   In a given case,
the circulation and temperature being favorably influenced by Aconite and Veratrum, Sulphite of
Soda exerts an immediate and marked controlling
influence over the fever poison.   Whilst if it had
been given without such preparation it would have
had no influence at all, or but slight influence.

Some causes of disease are destroyed and removed
by remedies that increase waste and excretion.   Preparations of Potash and Soda, especially the alka-

line diuretics act in this way. There are some organic remedies that exert a direct influence upon causes of disease, modifying or destroying them, as may be instanced in the action of Phytolacca in diphthéria. This action, however, in the majority of cases, is feeble.

Causes of disease acting in and from the blood, are frequently removed by stimulating the excretory organs. Some are removed principally by the skin, others by the bowels, others by the kidneys.

The cause of periodic disease, whatever it may be, plays a very important part in the diseases of some localities. Antagonize this cause, and the disease ceases, or at least is very much modified. Hence in the treatment of the diseases of the West, antiperiodics become the most important remedies.

Quinia is a true specific, and may be taken as the type of these remedies. It fails frequently, possibly it is administered nine times where its specific action is obtained once. But it is not the fault of the remedy, but of the doctor. If the diagnosis is correctly made, and the system is prepared for its administration, it will rarely fail, even when given in a single sufficient dose.

I am satisfied that the study of the direct antagonism of remedies to causes of disease, must advance the progress of rational medicine. It is possible, and I deem it probable, that such research will give us remedies controlling all zymotic disease in its early stage.

4. The human body is a complex structure, united

5

in functional activity by a nervous system. As this exerts a controlling influence, we should expect that its lesions would form a very important element of the study of pathology. This has not been the case, however, and we find pathologists and therapeutists giving it but very little attention. It is a wide field for study, and its cultivation will greatly advance medical science.

A few suggestions may not be out of place here:

Those functions which we have been accustomed to speak of as *vegetative*, are associated together, and to some extent governed by the ganglionic or sympathetic nervous system. It comprises digestion, blood-making, the circulation of the blood, nutrition, and secretion and excretion—these are the essentially vital functions, in the performance of which man has life. If they are properly performed, he has healthy life, if there is an aberration in either of them, one or more, he has diseased life. Is it possible to have disease, without a lesion of one of these? I think the reader will say it is not. If this be so, then this ganglionic system of nerves must play an important part in every disease.*

Control and association of these vital processes being in the ganglionic system of nerves, we would naturally expect it to furnish the readiest means of reaching them and correcting their lesions. If there are remedies then that influence the ganglionic nerves directly, and through them the vital

*See Principles of Medicine, page 306.

processes of the body, they must become our most direct and important therapeutic means. ' It is in this way that a large number of specific remedies act, as I believe. The sedatives, Aconite, Veratrum, Gelseminum, Lobelia, and others, as Cactus, Belladonna, Eryngium, Phytolacca, Hamamelis, Pulsatilla, etc., very certainly produce their effects through it.

The association of the spinal-cord with the sympathetic brings vital functions in relation with our conscious life, and through its superior expansion the brain, adds suffering from disease. Conversely, mal-conditions of conscious life are reflected through this association and influence vital processes.

Whilst, therefore, it is very important to reach lesions of vegetative life directly through the ganglionic system of nerves, it is no less important to control any disease producing influence that might be extended from the cerebro-spinal centres.

5. Lesions of waste and excretion are elements of every disease. In some they form a principal part, in others in less degree, but in all they require to be estimated in diagnosis and therapeutics. They range themselves under the common classification of excess, defect, and perversion, and usually it is not difficult to determine their character, and select means that exert a direct influence.

Constant waste is a necessity of life, as is constant removal of this waste. If the materials of the body are not broken down and removed as they have served their purpose, the body is old, imperfect, and

has lost functional power to this extent. If the
material is broken down and removed to the blood,
but not carried out by the excretions, we will have
an impairment of life from its presence in the
blood. I have given this subject full consideration
in my Principles of Medicine, pp. 116 to 185, to
which the reader is referred.

Too rapid waste of tissue is sometimes an important element of disease, requiring care in diagnosis
and the application of remedies.

A perversion in waste and excretion is a common
element of disease. In the breaking down of a
protean body, it passes through many phases, and
in its metamorphosis, it assumes forms that are
noxious to life, if they have any degree of perma-
nency, or are in any considerable quantity. Lesions
in *retrograde metamorphosis* are therefore to be estimated, and remedies which influence it become important.

We have already noticed that many causes of
disease act in and from the blood. They are zymotic poisons, or animal matter undergoing change,
and influence the blood and life in different degree,
in proportion to their quantity, and especially in
proportion to their activity in setting up the septic
process. These may be antagonized or destroyed
in many cases; in others the natural process of retrograde metamorphosis is stimulated, and they are
transformed into urea and other innocuous bodies
fitted for excretion by kidneys, skin and bowels.
Means that increase the activity of these excretions

are frequently sufficient for the removal of such causes of disease.

6. The necessity of regarding the nutritive processes during the progress of disease, is now admitted by all advanced physicians, and insisted upon by such writers as Chambers, Anstie, Bennett and others. Experience has conclusively proven that proper food with good condition of the digestive apparatus, without medicine, give a success in the treatment of the graver acute diseases, that was never obtained by any other method of treatment.

As we have already seen, the condition of the stomach and digestive apparatus is of *first* importance in all forms of disease, and its lesions demand *first* attention in our therapeutics. We have shown that this was essential to the successful administration of remedies, it is no less necessary that the patient may take and appropriate proper food.

The administration of remedies that increase functional activity of the digestive apparatus, or aid in the digestive process, are sometimes important means. The selection of appropriate food, and the use of restoratives is supplemental to this. The object is to place the digestive organs in good condition to receive and prepare food for admission to the blood; to furnish such material to the blood as may be necessary for its perfect organization, and for the renewal of tissue.

ABIES CANADENSIS.
(HEMLOCK.)

This agent has been employed in medicine for a long time—the bark in decoction as an astringent, the foliage in hot infusion as a diuretic and diaphoretic, and the oil as a stimulant local application. It undoubtedly possesses valuable properties. The following properties and uses are suggested to those who live where it may readily be obtained:

1st. A tincture of the recent *inner* bark in diluted alcohol; use in general asthenia with pallid mucous membranes, and feeble digestion: also, in diseases of the respiratory mucous membranes.

2nd. A tincture of the foliage in dilute alcohol; use in irritation of the urinary organs, and in disease of the skin.

ÆSCULUS GLABRA,
(BUCKEYE.)

Preparation.—Whilst the bark possesses medicinal properties in considerable degree, and may be used, a tincture of the nuts will probably be the best preparation.

Take of the recent nuts, fully ripened, four ounces; bruise them thoroughly, and cover with alcohol 76° one pint; let it stand for two weeks; strain and filter.

Of this tincture add from one to two drachms to four ounces of water—the dose being one teaspoonful.

The buckeye has been used to but a limited extent in medicine, yet its activity is such (as a poison), that it will probably prove very valuable when thoroughly studied. In my boyhood, I well remember persons carrying "buckeyes" in their pockets as a sovereign cure for "piles," and at a later period as a remedy for rheumatism. Doubtless this suggested the first use of the Æsculus in medicine.

It has been used in the treatment of hemorrhoids with much success, and I am satisfied that in some forms of the disease it is the most certain remedy we possess. I have also given it in a few cases of diseased uterus with good results—cases in which the entire organ was enlarged, the cervix tumid, with too frequent recurrence of the menstrual flow.

The marked influence of the Æsculus on the nervous system would suggest a line of experiment likely to lead to the development of valuable properties. It has already been employed as a stimulant to the nervous system in some cases of paralysis.

We may reason in this way: a remedy that cures hemorrhoids must exert a powerful influence upon the circulation; whilst its poisonous action, often witnessed — vertigo, diminished sight, wry neck, fixed eyes, paralysis, convulsions, etc., show its influence upon the nervous system.

ÆSCULUS HIPPOCASTANUM.
(HORSE CHESNUT.)

Preparation.—Take of the recent nut, fully ripe, four ounces, bruise it thoroughly, and cover with alcohol 76° one pint; let it stand fourteen days and filter.

Dose, two to four drops, in water.

The bark of this variety has been employed to a limited extent as a tonic, and possesses feeble antiperiodic powers. Quinine being employed to break the chill, this agent was sufficient to prevent its recurrence. The pulverized kernel has been used as a sternutatory for the relief of headache and facial neuralgia. The nuts were also thought to possess some special influence over hemorrhoids and rheumatism.

The influence upon the nervous system is similar in kind to the buckeye, though not so active. This probably will be its best field of action, standing midway between Belladonna on the one hand and Nux Vomica on the other.

It exerts the same influence upon the circulation as the Æsculus Glabra, and has been successfully employed in the treatment of hemorrhoids. It will doubtless be found to improve the circulation generally, and may be employed whenever there is want of power in the heart, capillary stasis, or tendency to congestion.

ACIDS.

There is a *specific* use for acids in the treatment of disease, which we wish to study carefully. In any form of disease we may have an excess of the alkaline salts of the blood. This may be the basis of diseased action, or but a complication rendering it more intense, but whether the one or the other, it needs to be recognized and have direct treatment.

The indications of excessive alkalinity are very plain, and need not be mistaken by the youngest practitioner. The color of the mucous membranes is *deep red*, especially of mouth and tongue; the coating of tongue, sordes, or any exudative material, has a dark color, usually brownish. It makes no difference what the diseased action is, in its totality, or what it is called, the *deep red*, somewhat *dusky* color always demands the administration of acids.

There is but one exception to this, and that is a rare one, in which the excess is of Soda, but with a defect of Potash. In this case the administration of a Salt of Potash will answer a better purpose than the Acid, or may be combined with it.

The Muriatic Acid is preferable in most acute cases, and should be used so diluted, and in such quantity, as to be pleasant to the patient, and until the indication for its use is removed. Lactic Acid is sometimes preferable with children, and in some

cases of chronic disease, especially when associated
with indigestion.   The vegetable Acids may be used
in acute disease, but are not so good as those
named.

ALKALIES.

It is well to consider the *specific* use of alkalies in
this relation; as they are the opposite of acids.
We may say of these, as of acids, that their deficiency is found as a constituent element in all forms
of disease—in some cases being the basis of a morbid action, in others but a complication; but, whenever found, an important element and demanding
direct treatment.

The symptoms of deficiency of these salts of the
blood are very plain, and, using the language of the
Prophet, "He who runs may read."   The tongue
is pallid and broad, its coating pasty and white, or
yellowish white.   The mucous membranes are uniformly pallid.   As these evidences are absolute and
readily determined, it is not necessary to name
others not so constant.

Whenever we find this deficiency of the alkaline
salts we will observe, as the result: loss of power
in the stomach, enfeebled digestion and slow absorption, impairment of the circulation, arrest of
nutrition and waste, and enfeebled innervation.
These will correspond in degree to the deficiency.

So marked are these results, that I have long regarded the diagnosis, with regard to excess or deficiency of the alkaline salts, as of the highest im-

portance. Indeed in some forms of disease, especially of a typhoid character, it is the principal element upon which a successful treatment is based.

Soda is the natural salt of the blood, and exists in the body in the largest proportion. Whenever, therefore, we have the evidence of deficiency of the alkaline salts, and no special symptoms indicating others we will give a Salt of Soda. In many cases I order Bicarbonate of Soda in water, in such quantity that it will make a pleasant drink, and let the patient have it freely.

If, at the same time, we wish an antiseptic influence, we may give the Sulphite or Hoposulphite of Soda or the Chloride of Sodium.

I am satisfied that I have seen patients die from deprivation of common salt during a protracted illness. It is a common impression that the food for the sick should not be seasoned, and whatever *slop* may be given, it is almost innocent of this essential of life. In the milk diet that I recommend in sickness, common salt is used freely, the milk being boiled and given hot. And if the patient can not take the usual quantity in his food, I have it given in his drink. This matter is so important that it can not be repeated too often, or dwelt upon too long.

The most marked example of this want of common salt I have ever noticed has been in surgical disease, especially in open wounds. Without a supply of salt the tongue would become broad, pallid, puffy, with a tenacious pasty coat, the effusion at the point of injury serous, with an unpleasant watery pus, which at last becomes a mere sanies or ichor. ~~A few days of a free allowance of salt~~ would change all this, and the patient would get along well.

A Salt of *Potash* is indicated where there is feebleness of the muscles to greater extent than can be accounted for by the disease. Occasionally such want is expressed in a marked manner by feebleness of the heart.

Ammonia will, occasionally, prove the best salt for temporary use, especially where there is great debility. But when so used, it should be followed by the free use of common salt, or some salt of soda.

ACHILLEA MILLEFOLIUM.
(YARROW.)

Preparation.— Prepare a tincture of the recent herb, ℥viij. to Alcohol 50° Oj. Dose, gtts. v. to ℈ss.

This agent, though feeble in its action, is much better than many in common use. It acts directly on the urinary apparatus, and the reproductive organs of the female. I have used it to allay irritation of the kidneys and vesical and urethral irritation. In these cases its influence is somewhat similar to Buchu and Uva Ursi. It is employed with advantage in atonic amenorrhœa, menorrhagia, and vaginal leucorrhœa.

ACONITUM NAPELLUS.
(ACONITE.)

Preparation.—A tincture of the root (imported from Germany) is the strongest and most uniform preparation. It should be prepared by percolation, the strength being ounce for ounce; though, if constantly made in the office, it will be easier to make it ʒviij. to the pint, the dose being proportionately increased.

The medium dose two-thirds of one drop, and the form of administration: ℞ Tincture of Aconite Root, gtts. x; Water, ʒiv.; a teaspoonful every hour in acute disease, every two or three hours in chronic disease. To a child two years old the proportion is gtts. v. to Water ʒiv.

Aconite is a stimulant to the sympathetic system of nerves, and increases the power of the heart to move the blood, at the same time that it places the blood-vessels in better condition for its passage. It will be recollected that the same system of nerves governs the movements of the heart and of the entire system of blood-vessels. What will influence one, therefore, will influence the other in the same manner.

But Aconite is said to be a sedative; and by a sedative we are to understand a remedy that diminishes the frequency of the pulse. How can Aconite, therefore, be a stimulant and a sedative?

There is no doubt but that Aconite is one of the most certain remedies we have to reduce the frequency of the pulse in certain conditions of disease. And the condition is that in which there is a want of power on the part of the heart, and a like want of innervation to the capillary system of blood-vessels. Aconite in small doses lessens the frequency of the pulse, because it removes obstruction to the free flow of blood in the vessels, and gives greater cardiac power.

We employ it in all forms of fever, to control the circulation, and diminish the temperature. Used in the doses named, it gives greater freedom to the circulation, at the same time that it diminishes the frequency of the pulse. It seems to remove obstruction to the free circulation of the blood, at the same time that it removes irritation of the cardiac nerves, and gives increased power to the heart.

Its action in inflammation is as pronounced as in fever. It directly antagonizes inflammatory action, and in the early stage will arrest it speedily—if this is the sedative indicated.

There are some diseases of an inflammatory character to which Aconite is *specific*, that deserve mention. The first of these is Tonsillitis, in which we employ it by internal administration, or better by the use of the steam atomizing apparatus. In some forms of mucous croup, with enfeebled circulation, in muco-enteritis, and in simple colitis or dysentery from cold, I never think of making any other prescription.

To point out the special indications for the use of Aconite I can not do better than reproduce the editorial in September *Journal* of 1868 on the "Differential Therapeutics of Veratrum and Aconite:"

To determine which of a class of remedies is applicable in a given case, is the most difficult task of the physician, and any information in this respect is of much value. I doubt whether any one using the two remedies named, would be willing to risk giving this estimate. Many may have an empirical intuition in regard to it, but most could venture nothing but a guess.

In general terms, Veratrum is the remedy in sthenia, Aconite in asthenia; but there are too many exceptions to this to make it a safe rule for our guidance.

Veratrum is the remedy where there is a frequent but free circulation. It is also the remedy where there is an active capillary circulation, both in fever and inflammation. A full and bounding pulse, a full and hard pulse, and a corded or wiry pulse, if associated with inflammation of serous tissues, call for this remedy.

Aconite is the remedy when there is difficulty in the capillary circulation, a dilatation and want of tonicity of these vessels, both in fever and inflammation.

It is the remedy for the frequent, small pulse, the hard and wiry pulse (except in the cases above named), the frequent, open and easily compressed pulse, the rebounding pulse, the irregular pulse, and indeed wherever there is the evidence of marked enfeeblement of the circulation.

It is the sedative I associate with Belladonna in congestion, especially of the nerve centers, and to relieve coma. Whilst I would use Veratrum with Gelseminum in determination of blood to the brain, and in active delirium.

Veratrum acts more efficiently upon the excretory organs; indeed I believe it to be one of the most certain remedies we have to increase excretion. Hence it is employed with great advantage for those purposes usually called alterative.

Aconite controls excessive activity of the excretory organs, whether of the bowels, kidneys or skin. Thus it is our most certain remedy in the summer complaint of children, associated with Belladonna in diabetes insipidus, with the bitter tonics and Strychnia in Phosphuria and Oxaluria, and with the mineral acids in night sweats.

ACTÆA ALBA.
(White Cohosh.)

Preparation. — Two preparations may be used: first, a tincture of the recent root, ℥viij. to Alcohol 76° Oj.; second, a tincture of the dried root in the same proportion, but using Alcohol of 98°. Let the dose range from one to twenty drops.

The White Cohosh has had but a limited use in medicine, yet it possesses such properties that it will undoubtedly prove useful when studied. The direction of experiment will be to determine its influence on the functions of waste and nutrition, and its special action on the reproductive organs of the female.

BLOOMINGTON, ILL., Sept. 30.

DR. SCUDDER: I intended to have written to you, in regard to one specific property of the *Actæa Alba*. As you have reached it in your order, you can do as you wish in regard to inserting this. It is specific in controlling after-pains. There is probably no remedy known that equals it. Make a tea of it, and drink freely. This power in controlling after-pains, suggests that it will prove invaluable in congestion and neuralgia of the womb.

W. FULTON, M. D.

AGAVE AMERICANA.
(CENTURY PLANT.)

The only report we have of this agent is from Dr. Penn, U. S. A., in the treatment of scurvy: "Every case has improved rapidly; the countenance, so universally dejected and despairing in the patient affected with scurvy, is brightened up by contentment and hope in two days from the time of its introduction. The most marked evidences of improvement were observable at every successive visit. From observing the effects of the Maguey in the cases which have occurred in this command, I am compelled to place it far above that remedy which, till now, has stood above every other—lime juice. The manner in which I use it is as follows: The leaves are cut off close to the root. They are placed in hot ashes until thoroughly cooked, when they are removed, and the juice expressed. The expressed juice is then strained, and given in doses of ʒij. to ʒiij. daily."

I should be glad if some of our southern readers would try a tincture of the recent leaves, made by cutting them in small pieces and covering with alcohol. We want to determine its influence on the circulation and on the nervous system. The dose would be about ten drops.

AGRIMONIA EUPATORIA.

Preparation.—Prepare a tincture from the fresh herb ʒviij. to Alcohol 50° Oj. Dose from gtts. j. to ʒss.

Agrimonia exerts a slight stimulant influence upon all the vegetative processes, and under its use we find an improvement of appetite, digestion and nutrition.

It exerts a specific influence upon mucous membranes, checking profuse secretion, and giving tone. Thus it has been employed with advantage in cases of chronic bronchitis, phthisis with increased secretion, and humoral asthma.

But it is especially useful in chronic catarrhal disease of the kidneys and bladder, and will frequently prove curative. It gives tone and strength to these organs, and may well replace the more common tonic diuretics in many cases.

ALETRIS FARINOSA.

The Aletris is a gastric stimulant and improves digestion. It has also proven a valuable tonic in uterine diseases. It is deserving a thorough examination, which I hope some of our readers will give it and report. Prepare a tincture from ʒviij. of the root to Alcohol 76° Oj. The dose would be from two to ten drops.

ALNUS RUBRA.
(Tag Alder.)

Preparation.—Prepare a tincture from the recent bark ʒviij. to Alcohol 50° Oj. Dose gtts. j. to xx.

We may employ the Alnus in infusion, or in the form of tincture with dilute alcohol; the first being preferable if we wish its greatest influence.

It exerts a specific influence upon the processes of waste and nutrition, increasing the one and stimulating the other. It is thus a fair example of the *ideal* alterative, and is one of the most valuable of our indigenous remedies.

Its special use seems to be in those cases in which there is superficial disease of the skin or mucous membranes, taking the form of eczema or pustular eruption. In these cases I have employed it as a general remedy, and as a local application with the best results. It does not seem to make much difference whether it is a phlyctenular conjunctivitis, an ulcerated sore mouth or throat, chronic eczema, or secondary syphilis presenting these characteristics, it is equally beneficial.

ALOES.

The use of Aloes in medicine should be quite limited, but still it has a place. I believe that in small quantity and in combination with other agents that act upon the upper intestinal canal, it proves a good cathartic, as in the following: ℞ Podophyllin, grs. x.; Leptandrin, grs. xxx.; Aloes, grs. xx.; Extract of Hyoscyamus, ℨss. Make thirty pills. One of them at night will prove an excellent laxative, and those who employ cathartics freely will like the formula.

But it is not for this purpose that I would recommend Aloes, but for one that may seem very singular. In small doses it exerts a direct influence upon the waste and nutrition of the nervous system. In cases of feeble innervation, especially in persons of gross habit, it will be one of our best agents. I have usually prescribed it with Tincture of Nux Vomica or with Tincture of Belladonna. The dose of a strong tincture being from two to ten drops.

In some cases it will prove serviceable when associated with the bitter tonics, as in this: ℞ Extract of Nux Vomica, grs. vj.; Aloes, grs. xv.; Hydrastine, ℨss. Make thirty pills. One may be given three or four times a day.

AMMONIUM, BROMIDE OF.

The Bromide of Ammonium is a stimulant to the nerve centers; increasing waste and improving nutrition.

I have employed it principally in epilepsy, in some cases of which it is undoubtedly a *specific*. I do not think I can point out the exact cases in which it is likely to prove curative, as the evidences of pathological states in this disease are very obscure. Its use, therefore, will have to be empirical.

I have used it now for some ten years, and it has given excellent satisfaction. But whilst it has effected permanent cures in a large number of cases, it has only proven of temporary benefit in some, and has wholly failed in others.

We not unfrequently meet with disease, in which there is disordered innervation, manifesting itself as epileptiform, partially spasmodic, or in other ways, but in which there is undoubtedly the same enfeeblement of the cerebro-spinal centers. In these cases Bromide of Ammonium is the remedy.

In diseases of children, I have been accustomed to employ this remedy in convulsions, following the first influence obtained by Lobelia or Gelseminum, and with marked success. When a child is subject to repeated attacks of convulsions from slight causes, the Bromide of Ammonium may be used to remove the predisposition.

In some cases of whooping cough it exerts a

direct action, as it does in many cases of nervous cough in both child and adult.

I have used it in this proportion : ℞ Bromide of Ammonium, ℥ss.; Water, ℥iv. A teaspoonful four times a day.

AMMONIUM, IODIDE OF.

Iodide of Ammonium increases retrograde metamorphosis at the same time that it exerts a stimulant influence upon the nervous system, especially the sympathetic system. Thus it can be employed with less risk than Iodide of Potassium, when the nutritive powers are feeble, as is the case occasionally in secondary syphilis.

It has been employed in certain cases of persistent headache with excellent results. They are those in which the eye is dull, the face expressionless, the circulation feeble, the patient being of a full habit. The dose will be: ℞ Iodide of Ammonium, ℨij.; Water, ℥iv. A teaspoonful every four hours.

AMPELOPSIS.

The Ampelopsis comes under the general classification of alteratives. It is a feeble agent in this direction and will have but a limited use. It would be well to have it thoroughly tested, and for this purpose I would suggest a tincture of the fresh bark, in doses of from one-fourth to one teaspoonful.

AMYGDALUS PERSICA.
(PEACH TREE.)

Preparation.—Thus far we have employed an infusion of the bark of the young limbs of the Peach Tree; and, to a limited extent, a tincture of the recent bark with dilute Alcohol. The first will·be found preferable in cases of acute gastric irritation; but for ordinary office use, I would suggest the following:

Take of the green bark of the young limbs (suckers), a sufficient quantity, and cover with Alcohol 50°, one pint to each eight ounces: let it stand for fourteen days, and express—a ·press of some kind will be an aid. The dose will be from five to thirty drops.

The infusion or tincture, as above prepared, has a direct influence in quieting irritation of the stomach and upper intestinal canal. It is also a mild tonic, improving the functions of digestion. For these purposes it is one of the most valuable articles in the Materia Medica.

It also exerts an influence upon the circulation, and upon the nervous system, which deserves investigation.

ANAGALLIS ARVENSIS.
(RED CHICKWEED.)

This agent possesses active properties, but has not been studied. It has been extolled in hydrophobia,

delirium, mania, epilepsy, etc., which will suggest
the line of experiment.

The best preparation, probably, will be a tincture
of the recent *Chickweed* in dilute Alcohol (50°),
℥viij. to the pint; dose quite small—coming within
one or two drops.

ANEMONE NEMOROSA.
(WOOD ANEMONE—WIND FLOWER.)

This is also an active agent, and will probably repay careful study. It influences the functions of
waste and repair, but acts directly upon the nervous
system. Belonging to the same family as the Pulsatilla, its action will be somewhat analogous.

The preparations best adapted for study will be a
tincture of the recent plant, made in the proportion
of ℥viij. to Alcohol 76° Oj.; using pressure to remove the fluid. It will be well to commence with
the fraction of a drop as a dose, say—℞ Tincture
of Anemone, gtts. x.; Water, ℥iv.; a teaspoonful
every two to four hours, gradually increasing as we
feel our way.

APOCYNUM CANNABINUM.
(INDIAN HEMP.)

Preparation.—The preparation I prefer is, an
alcoholic tincture, representing the crude article,
ounce for ounce. Of such fluid extract, the dose

will vary from the fraction of one drop to ten drops, as the maximum. If the physician prepares his tincture, it should be from the recently dried root, in the proportion of ℥viij. to Alcohol 76° Oj.

It is probable that the Apocynum Androsæmifolium possesses identical properties, and as the distinction is recognized with difficulty, even by those most conversant with botanic medicines, they have been used indiscriminately.

The Apocynum is a true *specific* for that atonic condition of the blood-vessels, that permits exudation, causing dropsy. I have employed it in my practice for some eight years, and it has not failed me in a single case, where the diagnosis was well made.

It is a positive remedy for dropsy, whether it takes the form of œdema, anasarca, or dropsy of the serous cavities, where there is no obstruction to the circulation, and no febrile action. We would not expect it to effect a cure in dropsy from heart disease, or ascites from structural disease of the liver, neither would we where there was a frequent, hard pulse, and other evidences of febrile action. Still in these cases, if we can partially remove the obstruction in the first case, and after an arrest of febrile action in the second, the Apocynum will remove the deposit.

It is not worth while to inquire how it removes dropsical accumulations. It seems to strengthen the circulation, and as absorption takes place there is an increased flow of urine.

7

I have also employed the Apocynum in cases of passive menorrhagia with advantage. It may be especially recommended in those cases in which the flow is constantly too profuse, too long, and too frequently repeated. I use it with water, in the following proportion: ℞ Fluid Extract of Apocynum, ℥j. to ℥ij.; Water, ℥iv.; a teaspoonful every three hours.

Latterly it has been used as an anti-rheumatic, with excellent results in some cases. With this, as with many other remedies, there are special symptoms indicating its use. If these are found in any disease, the remedy becomes specific. Thus in rheumatism, if there is a tendency to œdema, even slight puffiness of skin, or peculiar blanched glistening appearance, the Apocynum will be found a valuable remedy.

Following these indications I have used it with excellent results in some chronic diseases, especially where pain was a prominent symptom.

I have already spoken of it as a remedy for menorrhagia. It will also be found a valuable remedy in chronic metritis, with uterine leucorrhœa. In one case with profuse watery discharge from the uterus, it proved curative after other plans of treatment had failed.

ARALIA HISPIDA.
(DWARF ELDER.)

The Dwarf Elder has been extensively and successfully employed in dropsy. The infusion has usually been employed, and given freely.

I would suggest a tincture of the recent bark, in dilute Alcohol, in the proportion of ℥viij. to the Oj.; dose gtts. x. to ʒj.

I have employed it to but a limited extent, yet with good results. It has a very positive influence on the circulation, and upon secretion. Does it not act on them through the *sympathetic nervous system?* and may we not influence all the vegetative functions with it, as we do with some others? It is deserving thorough investigation.

ARNICA MONTANA.
(ARNICA.)

Preparation.—Prepare a tincture from the recent flowers, ℥viij. to Alcohol 76° Oj. Dose, the fraction of a drop.

It is not necessary to refer to the common local use of this agent, or discuss the question whether a tincture of Arnica is preferable to Alcohol alone as a local application. Every one has employed it in this way, and each has formed his own opinion. I think its local use valuable, but greatly over-estimated.

Can it be employed as an internal remedy with advantage? I am satisfied that it can. It is a valuable stimulant in many grave diseases where a stimulant is most required. But if used as a general stimulant, like Alcohol, it would be as apt to do harm as good.

It is a *specific* stimulant to the spinal nervous system, and will be found useful where there is want of innervation from this. I have seen most marked benefit from it in advanced stages of disease, where there was feeble respiratory power; difficulty of sleeping from impeded respiration; want of control over the excretion of urine and feces, etc.; evidences of impairment of spinal innervation. In such cases its beneficial influence may be noticed in a few hours.

I have frequently prescribed it for lame back, back-ache, and feelings of debility, soreness, etc., in the small of the back. It is only useful in those cases where there is feebleness, with deficient circulation; but in these the influence is direct and permanent.

Recently it has been employed in the treatment of pneumonia with good results. The cases reported, so far as I can learn, were asthenic with an enfeebled circulation. It was employed alone in doses of five to ten drops every three hours.

ARSENICUM.
(Arsenic.)

Arsenic is one of the agents that Eclectics have objected to, on the ground that it, like Mercury, was a depressant, and should be classified as an antiphlogistic. The use of Arsenic in the early part of this century, though limited, was in large and many times poisonous doses. Being a powerful excitant to the vegetative nerves, this use, if continued long, would produce a peculiar form of fever— "febris arsenicum"—with its attendant impairment of vital function. Finally, with impaired blood-making and nutrition, there would be developed arsenical dropsy, and in some rare cases death was the result.

This arsenical fever bears a very close resemblance to *quinism*, or *quinine poisoning*, in its symptoms, though there was not, in a majority of cases, such disturbance of the nervous system. There was also a difference in the termination, for whilst in quinism there was continued dryness of skin and scanty, high colored urine, and finally death from uræmia; in chronic poisoning by Arsenic there was finally a stage of relaxation, and though there was dropsy, the skin and kidneys acted freely.

We have long since determined that the mere matter of dose in medicine might be the difference between a poison and a remedy. If, for instance, we give one grain of Strychnia, we poison our pa-

tient, whilst if the dose had been but the fortieth
or thirtieth of a grain, it would have proven a vital
stimulant. If we administer five grains of Morphia,
the result is death; whilst a medicinal dose of one-
fourth of a grain would have produced refreshing
sleep. If we give large doses of Aconite, (say five
drops of a tincture of the root,) frequently repeated,
it increases the frequency of the pulse, impairs the
circulation, and irritates the nervous system. But,
in medicinal doses, it lessens the frequency of the
pulse, gives freedom to the circulation, and relieves
irritation of the nervous system. If we give large
doses of Veratrum, it impairs the circulation,
arrests vital processes, and produces death; whilst
medicinal doses give increased freedom to the
circulation and diminish the frequency of the
pulse.

It seems strange to me that these things have not
had due consideration, and that the remedial action
of drugs has not been kept distinct from their
poisonous effects when given in large doses. We
have already seen, that the dose of medicine should
be the smallest quantity that will give the desired
influence, and that in a rational system of medicine,
its influence should always be to restore normal
function, and not as a disturbing element.

There is another view of this subject which is
important in this consideration. A drug which
may be poisonous in health, or in some conditions
of disease, will be curative in other conditions of
disease. Thus we regard the disease as antagoniz-

ing the remedy, quite as much as the remedy antagonizes the disease, and the influence is toward the restoration of healthy function. Give a healthy man almost any of our common medicines, and after a time he will become diseased, the disease being of that kind and of that part that the medicine cures. Thus, if we give Quinine to cure malarial fever, its influence is kindly, but if there is no malarial disease, it causes irritation of the nervous system. If we give Belladonna when there is an enfeebled capillary circulation, the influence is kindly and curative, but it is the reverse if we already have capillary spasm.

This is especially the case with the more powerful remedies, with which Arsenic should be classed, and they should never be employed unless the symptoms indicating them are very distinct.

Such a brief statement of facts I have deemed necessary in this case, on account of the prejudice of our School to these agents—a prejudice which grew out of their abuse. This prejudice is so strong now, that one hardly dare risk making a study of the tabooed articles, and yet common honesty demands that it be done.

In *small* doses, and when indicated, Arsenic may be regarded as a vital stimulant, and one of the most powerful of this class. But we must not forget that the dose *must* be small, and there *must* be special indications for its use. What are these indications?

In that condition of the blood, and of nutrition,

where there is a tendency to the deposit of a low or imperfect albuminoid material — yellow tubercle, caseous deposits—or degeneration of tissue, Arsenic may be used as a blood-maker, and especially to improve nutrition.

A class of skin diseases depending upon such deposits, or an enfeebled nutrition, is cured by Arsenic. Among these are the more chronic affections—the squamæ, the chronic vesiculæ, some of the pustulæ, and the tuberculæ. It will not cure all cases, it will do harm if injudiciously used, but it affords relief in many otherwise intractable.

But, it should never be employed where there is irritability of the nerve centers, and especially of the sympathetic. This rule I think is absolute, and must be constantly regarded. Arsenic is a *nerve-stimulant;* quite as much so as phosphorus, with this addition—that its action is greatly intensified when there is already erythism of the nerve centers.

It has been successfully employed in some cases of phthisis, presenting the condition above named. Prof. Howe uses it in combination with Veratrum, and there is no doubt that this renders the system tolerant of Arsenic where it could not otherwise be employed.

Arsenic is topically employed to destroy malignant growths. The majority of the "cancer specialists" use it in some form, and their preparations differ only in the inert material with which it is combined. The preparation now employed most frequently is made as follows: Take Hydrated Sesquioxide of Iron a sufficient quantity, throw it on a paper filter, and when of the consistence of an ointment, add an equal part of Lard. To this add Arsenious Acid, in the proportion of ʒss. to ʒj. to the ounce.

Arsenic may be employed in the treatment of some cases of intermittent fever with excellent results. They are those marked by impairment of sympathetic innervation, and with a general want of nervous excitability. The dose should be very small, gtts. v. to x. of Fowler's Solution to ℥iv. of Water; a teaspoonful every two or three hours. I have used the Homœopathic pellets, medicated with Fowler's Solution, and though the dose was not more than the twentieth to the one-hundredth of a drop, the effect was marked, where specially indicated.

It is also used with advantage in atonic diarrhœa, with indigestion, the conditions being as above named. Especial benefit has been observed in those cases in which there were periods of great depression, followed by hectic fever.

I need hardly say in conclusion, that Arsenic is one of those agents that will do either good or harm. Good if given in a proper case, and in medicinal doses; harm if not indicated by special symptoms, or contra-indicated as above named, or if given in poisonous doses.

Fowler's Solution is the preparation to be preferred. Dose from the fraction of a drop to two drops.

ARTEMESIA ABSINTHIUM.
(WORMWOOD.)

Preparation.—For experiment, I would suggest a tincture with dilute Alcohol, 76°, in the proportion of ℥viij. to the pint; vary the dose from one drop to one drachm.

This agent has been used principally as a vermifuge, but lately it has given place to the Chenopodium, and to Santonine. It possesses very decided medicinal properties, however, and deserves a thorough examination. It influences the nervous system, especially the sympathetic.

ARTEMESIA SANTONICA.
(WORMWOOD.)

We only wish to consider the crystallizable principle—Santonine—here. Its principal use has been as a vermifuge in cases of ascaris lumbricoides, for which it has been found quite efficient. But in using it for this purpose many have noticed that it exerted a peculiar influence upon the brain, and upon the eyes—rendering objects blue, yellow, or green; and that it passed off in the urine, giving it a peculiar color.

It exerts a *specific* action upon the bladder and urethra, stimulating contraction of the first, and allaying irritation of the second. It is especially valuable in cases of retention of the urine in children during protracted disease; in doses of half to one grain, it is prompt and certain. I have also employed it to relieve irritation of the urethra, especially in women suffering from uterine disease, and with good success.

Its influence upon the nervous system needs to be studied. I judge it to be a nerve stimulant, and have employed it for this purpose to a limited extent.

ASCLEPIAS.
(SILKWEED.)

Preparation. — The best preparation for experiment will be a tincture of the recent root, in the proportion of ℥viij. to Alcohol 76° Oj.; note its effect in small as well as large doses.

The A. Incarnata, A. Syriaca, etc., deserve a careful investigation. In weak infusion they all prove diaphoretic, and to some extent diuretic. It is claimed by those who have made considerable use of them, that they stimulate all the secretions.

ASCLEPIAS TUBEROSA.
(PLEURISY ROOT.)

Preparation.—Whilst I prefer a tincture made as above, I have used the alcoholic fluid extract of the dried root, made to represent ounce for ounce; the dose being from one drop for a child two years old, to ten drops for an adult.

It is especially a child's remedy, being feeble in action, though quite certain. When given freely, it is one of the most certain diaphoretics we have, providing the pulse is not frequent, and the temperature increased. Even in the small dose of one drop, following the use of the special sedatives, it will markedly increase *true* secretion from the skin.

Recollect that there is a difference between sweating and secretion. There may be a profuse exudation of water, the surface being bathed in perspiration, and yet but little secretion. Excretion by the skin is a vital process, and takes place by means of secreting cells. It goes on best where the skin is soft and moist, and not when covered with drops of sweat.

I employ Asclepias in diseases of children, believing that it allays nervous irritability, is slightly sedative, and certainly increases secretion from the skin. I use it with Veratrum and Aconite, in febrile and inflammatory diseases, and in mild cases, very frequently give it alone. Bear in mind that it is a feeble remedy and too much must not be expected.

ASPIDIUM FILIX MAS.
(MALE FERN.)

This agent is only used as a vermifuge, especially for the removal of the tapeworm. For this purpose the Ethereal Oil is used in doses of twenty drops to one drachm.

ASAFŒTIDA.

Whilst I think but little of the fœtid gum as an antispasmodic, I regard it as a valuable gastric stimulant, and also as a nerve stimulant. In nervous dyspepsia, especially, it will be found valuable. The following is a good form: ℞ Asafœtida, ℨss.; Hydrastine, ℨss.; Aloes, grs. x. Make thirty pills, and give one three times a day. As a nerve stimulant I have used: ℞ Extract of Nux Vomica, grs. x.; Asaf., grs. xl. Make twenty pills, and give one at night.

ATROPA BELLADONNA.
(BELLADONNA.)

Preparation.—Whilst for some purposes a solution of the Alkaloid Atropia will prove the best preparation, I prefer, for general use, an alcoholic tincture of the recent plant, representing the crude article ounce for ounce. Of this the maximum dose will be one drop, but frequently one-fifth to one-half of this will serve a better purpose.

For hypodermic use, we employ a solution of Atropia, in the proportion of one grain to the ounce of distilled water. The dose would be five to ten drops. This is also the best proportion for use to dilate the pupil. As a collyrium, we would add ℨj. of this solution to ℥j. of distilled water.

The *specific* use of Belladonna is as a stimulant to the capillary circulation, especially of the nerve centers—a remedy opposed to congestion. My attention was first drawn to it by an article from Brown-Sequard, giving the results of his experiments with the drug, stating that with the microscope he had seen marked contraction of the capillaries following its use. It at once suggested itself to me, that if it would cause capillary contraction, it would be *the* remedy for congestion ; and I at once commenced experimenting with it in this direction.

I well recall my first marked case : a boy about eight years old, suffering from malignant rubeola. The entire surface was swollen and dusky ; the eyes dull ; the pupils dilated ; the face expressionless ; breathing labored, and wholly unconscious for forty-eight hours. The administration of Belladonna alone (in small doses) was sufficient to restore consciousness, and a free circulation, with good appearance of the eruption, in twenty hours.

The evidences in its favor rapidly accumulated, so that in eighteen months I used it with a feeling of almost certainty for this purpose.

Whilst it exerts the same influence on all persons, and at all ages, the true pathological condition being determined, it is especially valuable in treating diseases of children. In the young, the immature nervous centers suffer more severely, and we find the opposite conditions, of irritation with determination of blood, and atony with congestion.

The symptoms calling for the use of Belladonna are usually very plain : the patient is dull and stupid—and the child drowsy, and sleeps with its eyes partly open; the countenance expressionless; the eyes are dull, and the pupils dilated, or immobile; whilst, as it continues, respiration becomes affected, and the blood imperfectly aerated.

In these cases I prescribe Belladonna: in the adult, in the proportion of gtts. x. to gtts. xx., to Water ℥iv.; in the child gtts. v. to ℥iv.; in each a teaspoonful every hour. As these are mostly febrile cases, or at least have a feeble, frequent circulation as an element, I give Aconite in the usual doses.

Belladonna is also a *specific* in incontinence of urine. Not that it will cure any case, but those in which an enfeeblement of the pelvic circulation is the principal cause. Probably a lesion of the spinal cord has also much to do with it. Of course, it gives no relief where the incontinence arises from vesical irritation. The dose in this case will be the same as above named, but only repeated four times a day.

Belladonna is also a *specific* in *diabetes insipidus;* even a Belladonna plaster across the loins being sufficient in many cases for its arrest.

Belladonna is undoubtedly a *prophylactic* against scarlatina, as I have thoroughly proven in my practice. Recollect, however, that it is only prophylactic in small doses; in doses sufficient to produce dilatation of the pupil it has no such influence.

Belladonna has other special uses, but they may be briefly summed up: if in any case there is an enfeebled circulation, with stasis of blood, Belladonna is the remedy. Of course, acting upon some parts more directly than others, its influence will be more decided, but there is no case, with condition as above, in which it will not be beneficial.

I may say in conclusion, that we want a *good* preparation of the recent herb; and then it *must* be used in small doses to obtain the influences named. The doses given are the *maximum*. As we have had occasion to say before, the druggists care little about the quality of medicines sold; they are simply articles of merchandise, and there is little, if any, professional *esprit* with them, to aid us in having them good. Therefore every physician must be on his guard when purchasing, and had better buy of first hands, and of those of proven honesty.

APIS MELLIFICA.
(Honey Bee.)

The Honey Bee possesses marked medicinal properties, but from a prejudice against such remedies, has been but little employed.

An infusion of twelve to twenty Honey Bees in a pint of boiling water, is one of the most certain diuretics I have ever employed in cases of suppression of urine from atony. It is also a very efficient remedy in retention of urine, and in some cases of irritation of the urethra.

I have used a tincture for the same purpose, and also for inflammation of subcutaneous structures, with tensive and lancinating pains, and in irritation of the skin. I have prepared my own tincture, in the proportion of ℈j. to Alcohol 98° Oj. Dose one to two drops.

I have seen a number of cases of disease in women characterized by sensations of heat, and burning pains in the bladder and course of the urethra, with frequent desire to micturate. These have been promptly relieved by the use of Tincture Apis, and in two cases of chronic disease of long standing, a permanent cure was effected, following the relief of these unpleasant symptoms.

AGARIC.*

HISTORY.—This is obtained from various fungus plants of the mushroom tribe. They absorb a great amount of oxygen with evolution of hydrogen and carbonic acid gas, and contain considerable proportions of nitrogen. They are destructive to nearly all organic matter upon which they grow. According to Dr. M. A. Curtis, of N. C., the genus boletus, as now constituted, includes only fleshy species, with a hymenium composed of *sporable tubes*. Those species formerly included in Boletus, and whose hymenium is composed of *pores*, now form the genus Polyporus.

The *Polyporus Officinalis* (*Boletus Laricis*), known by the name of *White Agaric*, *Purging Agaric*, etc., is procured from Asia, Corinthia, Russia, Central America, and the Rocky Mountains, where it is found growing upon the Larch. It is in masses,

*The following is taken from the new edition of King's American Dispensatory.

varying from the size of an ordinary apple to that of a large nutmeg-melon; its shape somewhat resembles a horse's hoof; it is reddish-gray or yellow externally, whitish internally, and of a spongy, friable consistence; *hymenium* concrete; *substance of the pileus* consisting of subrotund pores, with their simple dissepiments; *pileus* corky-fleshy, ungulate, zoned, smooth; *pores* yellowish; it has a feeble odor, and a bitter, acid, somewhat sweetish taste. Braconnot found in it 72 parts resinous matter, 2 bitter extractive, 26 of a nutritious animalized principle, which he termed *fungin*. Benzoic acid and several salts have likewise been found in it. It is collected in August and September, deprived of its outer covering, and then dried and placed in the sun.

The *Polyporus* (*Boletus*) *Ignarius, Agaric of the Oak,* is a fungus found on the oak, cherry, willow, plum, and other trees; when young it is soft, but gradually becomes hard and woody. In shape it somewhat resembles the preceding; its upper smooth surface is marked with dark circular ridges, and its under is very porous, and of a yellowish-white color. It is tasteless and inodorous. The *Polyporus* (*Boletus*) *Fomentarius,* growing on similar trees with the *P. Ignarius,* when cut in slices, beaten, soaked in a solution of nitre, and dried, forms an inflammable substance, known as *Spunk, Amadou,* or *German Tinder.* The *Polyporus Pinicola* grows upon the pine, birch, tamarac, fir, and similar trees; with absolute alcohol the fresh fungus forms a dark-red,

intensely bitter tincture. A white amorphous powder, called *laricin*, is obtained from some of these
plants. It has a bitter taste, is soluble in alcohol
and oil of turpentine, forms a paste with boiling
water, and has the formula $C_{14}H_{12}O_4$.

PROPERTIES AND USES. — The dust of the *Larch
Agaric* is irritating to mucous surfaces, causing
tears when it enters the eyes, and sneezing, cough,
and nausea, when the nostrils are exposed to it.
It has been used in half-drachm or drachm doses
as a purgative; in larger doses as an emetic. In
doses of from three to ten grains, gradually increasing to sixty grains in the course of the twenty-
four hours, it has been found efficacious in arresting
the nocturnal perspiration of consumptives. Externally, it has been used, together with the *Agaric
of the Oak*, as a styptic, and said to restrain not only
venous but arterial hemorrhages, without the use of
ligatures. It does not appear, however, to possess
any real styptic power, or to act otherwise than
dry lint, sponge, or other soft applications. Prepared with nitre, as for tinder, it has been used as a
species of moxa.

The *P. Officinalis* and the *P. Pinicola*, in doses of
from three or four grains of the powder, repeated
every three or four hours, or of the concentrated
tincture in doses of five drops, have both been found
valuable in the cure of obstinate and long standing
intermittents, and other diseases common to malarial districts; as, obstinate bilious remittent fever,
chronic diarrhœa, chronic dysentery, periodical neu-

ralgia, nervous headache, ague cake, and increased flow of urine. They have likewise proved useful in long standing jaundice, and in the chills and fever common among consumptive patients.

The tincture of Boletus exerts a marked influence upon the spinal and sympathetic nervous system, in certain cases of disease. It has been successfully employed in the treatment of epilepsy and chorea, and to check the rapid pulse with hectic fever and night sweats in phthisis. It has also been recommended in insanity where there is a feeble cerebral circulation and imperfect nutrition. And, also, in neuralgia, with similar symptoms.

BAPTISIA TINCTORIA.

Preparation.—The Baptisia has been principally employed in infusion, and I am well satisfied that this is the best preparation for general use. Still, as it will be inconvenient in many cases, I would recommend in addition, a tincture by percolation, using ℥viij. of the ground bark to Oj. of Alcohol of 76°. Of an infusion of ℥j. to ℥iv. of boiling water, the dose is one teaspoonful; of the tincture as named, ℥ij. to Water, ℥iv., dose, a teaspoonful.

With some the Baptisia has been a favorite remedy for sore mouth and sore throat, using it locally, and for this purpose it is one of the most valuable remedies we have. I judge, however, that if you should ask, in what particular variety of sore mouth or throat it was found best? you would have difficulty in getting an answer.

It is in those cases in which there is enfeebled capillary circulation, and tendency to ulceration, that it is *specific*. That is, the condition is one of atony, with tendency to molecular death and decomposition. The remedy is, therefore, stimulant and antiseptic.

It may be employed with the greatest certainty in any form of sore mouth or throat presenting the characteristics named. Especially in stomatitis ulcerata, or cancrum orris, in cynanche maligna, and in the sore throat of scarlatina maligna; but it is not only a good local application in these cases, but a most valuable internal remedy.

It is *specific* to the condition upon which such sore mouth and throat is based, whether it is manifested in this way, or in ulceration of Peyer's follicles in typhoid fever. Thus I have employed it with very marked advantage, in all cases showing putrescency, and tendency to softening and breaking down of tissue.

It is not a remedy for acute inflammation, whether erythematous or deep seated, and in ordinary stomatitis or cynanche, it is not a remedy. In diphtheria presenting acute inflammatory symptoms, it is worse than useless. But in diphtheria with swollen and enfeebled mucous membranes, dusky or livid discoloration, or blanched appearance, with tendency to ulceration and sloughing, there is no remedy more certain.

I have successfully employed the Baptisia in *typhoid* dysentery, as have others. But as will be seen, this is but the condition named above for its specific action. So long as there is an acute inflammation, with stools of blood or pure mucus, this is not beneficial, but when the discharges resemble "prune juice, the washing of meat, or are muco-purulent," with general symptoms of an analogous character, then it becomes one of our most certain remedies.

BENZOIC ACID.

I prefer to use Benzoic Acid in solution in Alcohol, ʒj. to the Oj. to the tincture of Benzoin, though the latter will answer the purpose. The dose will vary from ten to sixty drops, according to the effect desired.

Its first use is in irritable bladder, with deposits of uric acid or triple phosphates; in either case its use will prove beneficial.

Its second use is in irritation of the sympathetic and spinal system of nerves, with uric acid deposits.

Its third use is as a stimulant to the brain in cases of exhaustion with Phosphuria. I have used it in this case alternated with a preparation of Phosphorus—either the Phosphuretted Oil or the Tincture—with advantage. These are usually cases of exhaustion from over-exertion of the mind, as frequently met with among our business men.

BERBERIS VULGARIS.
(BARBERRY.)

A tincture of the recent bark, in the proportion of 3viij. to Alcohol 76° Oj., is suggested. Dose varying from ten drops to one drachm.

Will some of our Eastern practitioners give us their experience with this agent; or if it has not been employed alone, will some one test it thoroughly. Evidently it has an influence upon the gastro-intestinal mucous membrane, and probably on associate viscera.

BEBEERINÆ SULPHAS.

This is not the so-called Berbeerin from the Berberis Vulgaris, but a well-defined salt from the Nectandra Rodiæi. As found in commerce, it is in glittering scales of a brownish-yellow color, and when triturated forms a yellowish powder.

It exerts a specific action upon the uterus, but thus far it has been principally employed in cases of menorrhagia. In this case its influence is very marked, controlling the hemorrhage, and preventing its recurrence. As we have other remedies for the milder cases, its use might be confined to those in which there is profuse discharge at each menstrual period, and where they recur too frequently. The dose will be from two to three grains every three or four hours.

BISMUTH.

We employ Bismuth in two forms. The sub-nitrate in doses of from one to two grains; the liquor Bismuth (solution of Citrate of Bismuth), in doses of from gtts. x. to ℥j.

The first use of Bismuth is to allay irritation of the gastro-intestinal mucous membrane; and for this purpose it has been extensively employed. Usually the sub-nitrate in impalpable powder, is employed in small doses frequently repeated for gastric irritation, and in doses of five to ten grains for intestinal irritation, with diarrhœa.

The second may be called its *specific* use, for chronic gastro-intestinal irritation, or dyspepsia with diarrhœa. Here I employ the Liquor Bismuth in doses of from a half to one teaspoonful four times a day. In inveterate cases, not amenable to treatment, and of years duration, I have had the happiest results.

I have omitted to name the common use of Bismuth for water-brash, in some cases of which it is very effectual.

The powdered sub-nitrate is also the most effectual local application for irritation of the skin—*chafing*—either in the infant or adult. For this purpose. the part is thoroughly dusted, and it is repeated as often as necessary to keep it dry.

BROMINE.

Bromine is not employed as an internal remedy, though its salts have been used largely within the last ten years. It may be employed with advantage as an inhalation in croup and diphtheria, and as a stimulant in phthisis. For croup it has been used in the proportion of ten drops to two ounces of water.

BROMIDE OF POTASSIUM.

Bromide of Potash is a very greatly overestimated remedy. When I commenced practice it was only used in cases of spermatorrhœa to relieve sexual irritation—now it is recommended for every nervous ill that flesh is heir to.

I think it has one *specific* use, and that is as a remedy for epilepsy when associated with irritation of the reproductive organs, or especially in irritation of the cerebellum. In such cases I have used it with much success. The dose will be about twenty grains three times a day.

I only use it in spermatorrhœa, in those cases in which the person is of a plethoric habit, with great venereal excitement — cases approximating satyriasis, rather than spermatorrhœa. In these I administer it in doses of thirty to sixty grains at bedtime.

9

BIDENS BIPINNATA—CONNATA—FRONDOSA.
(SPANISH NEEDLES.)

Preparation.—Prepare the tincture from the recent herb, in the proportion of ℥viij. to Alcohol 76° Oj., using pressure. Dose from five to thirty drops.

The different varieties of Bidens deserve investigation. Reference to the Dispensatory or Materia Medica will give the direction it should take. I am especially interested in the action of the B. Frondosa on the heart and circulation.

BRYONIA.

We employ the German tincture of Bryonia in the proportion of gtts. v. to gtts. xxx. to water ℥iv.; a teaspoonful every one, two, or three hours.

I have experimented with the Bryonia for some ten years, but without satisfactory results until lately. During the past winter I have treated some cases in which the remedy was a true specific. The most marked symptom indicating its use, that I have noticed, is a dusky flushing of the cheeks, especially over the right malar. Pain in the right side of the face and head, burning in eyes and nose, with acrid nasal discharge. The pulse is full and hard, urine scanty, and bowels constipated. With the first symptom named I should prescribe it in any form of disease, though it is used most frequently in rheumatism, pneumonia and catarrhal affections.

CALX.
(LIME.)

Lime is used for the ordinary purpose of an antacid, and in some cases is preferable to any other alkali. This is especially the case in indigestion, with the formation of lactic acid from decomposing food. Here there is not unfrequently an excess of the normal salts of the blood, and we can not use the salts of soda and potash to neutralize gastric acidity. It may be stated, as a general rule, that it will be found beneficial in cases of infantile dyspepsia, and in dyspepsia of the adult, with acid eructations during digestion.

Its *specific use* is in cases of furunculus or boils, and other inflammations of cellular tissue, terminating in suppuration. Why it has this specific influence I do not propose to say, but the fact I have proven in scores of cases. Given a case in which boils are being continually developed, the use of lime water will effect a radical cure. It is given in doses of a wineglassful three or four times a day.

CAMPHOR.

Camphor in small doses is a stimulant, in large doses a sedative, to the nervous system. I do not regard it as having a very extended use in medicine, though for the purpose named, it may sometimes be employed with advantage. In low forms of dis ease, with insomnia and restlessness, I have used it alone, and in combination with stimulant doses of Opium or Morphia, and Quinine.

As a topical stimulant, it may be employed with advantage, when the integrity of the part is threatened from enfeebled circulation.

CANNABIS SATIVA.
(HEMP).

The tincture of Cannabis should be prepared from the recent wild plant whilst in flower, but as we can not get this, we use a tincture prepared from the *churrus*, a species of extract from the recent plant, imported from India. The dose will vary from one to five drops.

In small doses it is stimulant to the cerebro-spinal centers; in large doses it produces intoxication, and finally arrest of function. It exerts an influence upon the urinary and reproductive apparatus that may be rendered available in practice, and also to some extent upon the skin.

I have employed the Cannabis *specially* to relieve irritation of the kidneys, bladder and urethra. It will be found especially beneficial in vesical and urethral irritation, and is an excellent remedy in the treatment of gonorrhœa.

I do not like it as a remedy for intemperance, (chronic alcoholism), so well as a combination of Nux Vomica and Iodine, with a bitter tonic; though in some cases it may be used with marked advantage, and the habit finally broken up by its use.

CANTHARIS VESICATORIA.
(Spanish Fly.)

I object to the use of the blister, as a means of counter-irritation, and going further than this, I object to counter-irritation as a means of cure, when it can possibly be avoided, and I think it may be avoided in nearly all cases.

As an internal remedy, Cantharis will have but one use—as a stimulant to the urinary apparatus, especially the bladder. For this purpose it may be employed in small doses.

CACTUS GRANDIFLORUS.
(Night-Blooming Cereus.)

Preparation.—We prepare a tincture from the recent plant, in the proportion of ℥iv., to Alcohol 98° Oj. The dose will vary from one to ten drops.

The influence of Cactus seems to be wholly exerted on the sympathetic nervous system, and especially upon, and through the cardiac plexus. It does not seem to increase or depress innervation, (neither stimulant, nor sedative,) but rather to influence a regular performance of function. I am satisfied, however, that its continued use improves the nutrition of the heart, thus permanently strengthening the organ. It has a second influence, which is of much importance to the therapeutist. It exerts a direct influence upon the circulation and nutrition of the brain, and may thus be employed with advantage in some diseases of this organ. We can see very readily how this may be. The cardiac nerves are derived from the upper part of the sympathetic, and judging from the anatomy of the part, the first cervical ganglion being the principal nervous mass in the cervical region, must furnish innervation through the cardiac nerves, as it certainly controls the circulation and nutrition of the brain.

The Cactus is a *specific* in heart disease, in that it gives strength and regularity to the innervation of the organ. Its influence is permanent, in that it influences the waste and nutrition of the organ, increasing its strength. It exerts no influence upon the inflammatory process, and hence is not a remedy for inflammatory disease.

Feelings of weight and pressure at the præcordia, difficult breathing, fear of impending danger, etc., are at once removed. Such irregularity of action, whether violent, feeble, or irregular, as is dependent upon the innervation, is readily controlled. Thus, in the majority of cases of *functional* heart disease it gives prompt relief, and, if continued, will effect a cure. In those cases in which there is another lesion acting as a cause, as in some gastric, enteric, or uterine lesions, these must receive attention, and be removed to make the cure radical.

In structural heart disease, the first use of remedies is to relieve the distressing sensation in the region of the heart, and the unnatural fear of danger which attends them. As these spring from disordered innervation, in the majority of cases, the Cactus gives prompt relief. As we have seen above, its continuance favors normal waste and nutrition, as well as regular action. Hence, its continued use is followed by the removal of adventitious tissue; and an increase in the strength of its contractile fibre. Hence, it is really curative in many cases of structural heart disease.

I have some cases on my case book, of such aggravated form, that no one would believe they could live a twelvemonth; yet, after a lapse of five years, they are enjoying comfortable health.

But it will not relieve or cure cases of valvular deficiency, dilatation of the openings of the heart, or fatty degeneration. It is well, in estimating its action, to bear this in mind.

In its influence upon the nervous system, it more nearly resembles Pulsatilla; giving relief in that condition known as nervousness. But farther than this, it gives regularity of cerebral function, and permanently improves nutrition of the nervous centers.

CAPSICUM.
(CAYENNE PEPPER.)

Capsicum is a powerful topical stimulant; but its general influence is feeble. As Capsicum, it never gains admission to the circulation, and, in the process of digestion, it almost wholly loses its properties as a remedy.

Capsicum is used as a topical stimulant to the skin, and with advantage where the circulation is feeble, and there is need of such stimulation. It also exerts the revulsive influence of other rube-facients.

Its influence, when taken into the stomach, is of the same character. It excites the nerves, and calls an increased flow of blood to the part. In torpid states of the gastric mucous membrane, such action may be very desirable, may even be essential to life: as, in congestive intermittent. It is the topical action upon the gastric mucous membrane that is beneficial in some cases of delirium tremens.

The solar plexus, the most important of the vegetative nerve centers, may be thus influenced from the stomach. The stimulant influence of Capsicum may, therefore, be extended through this, and be of marked advantage in states of great and sudden prostration with tendency to congestion.

CARBO-LIGNI.
(WOOD CHARCOAL.)

Is an absorbent and antiseptic, and has this general use, both internally and topically. Given in water-brash, or where there is decomposition of the food, it is sometimes quite beneficial. So in topical disease—with free secretion and tendency to sepsis—its local application absorbs the one and checks the other.

The *specific* use of charcoal is to arrest hemorrhage from the bowels. It is used in enema, ℥j. to ℥ij. finely powdered, to four ounces of water, thrown

up the rectum. Why it checks it I can not tell;
that it does it, I have the evidence of my own eyes.

CASSIA ACUTIFOLIA.
(SENNA.)

Senna is a 'mild cathartic; but its action is frequently attended with much tormina, and to some
is very unpleasant. As it does not increase elimi-
nation by the bowels, its use as a cathartic is quite
limited, and it may well be replaced by other
remedies.

It exerts, however, a special influence in colic,
which renders it an important remedy. We have
generally employed it in the form of the Compound
Powder of Jalap and Senna, in doses of five or ten
grains, frequently repeated until relief is obtained.
An infusion of Senna—or the tincture will answer
the same purpose—for the relief of colic, whether
the common wind-colic or that known as bilious, I
regard as one of our best remedies.

CAULOPHYLLUM.
(BLUE COHOSH.)

We employ this remedy in infusion as a parturient, and in the form of a tincture of the recently
dried root, ℥viij. to Alcohol 76° Oj. The alcoholic
fluid extract, representing ounce for ounce, is also a
good preparation.

Caulophyllum exerts a very decided influence

upon the parturient uterus, stimulating normal contraction, both before and after delivery. Its first use, in this case, is to relieve false pains; its second, to effect co-ordination of the muscular contractions; and third, to increase the power of these. The first and second are the most marked, yet the third is quite certain. Still if any one expects the marked influence of Ergot, in violent and continued contractions, he will be disappointed.

I judge that it exerts its influence through the hypogastric plexus; though to some extent it influences every process controlled by the sympathetic. Acting in this way it influences the circulation, nutrition, and functions of the reproductive organs. I have employed it in chronic uterine diseases with some advantage; but further study is necessary to point out the particular cases.

It may be used with good effect in some cases of nervous disease; especially in that condition known as *asthenic plethora*.

As a remedy for rheumatism it is inferior to the Macrotys, but in some cases it exerts a better influence. My experience has not been sufficient to point out these cases, and in this respect the remedy needs further study.

I would suggest, also, the trial of a tincture of the *recent* root.

CEANOTHUS AMERICANUS.
(REDROOT.)

This agent deserves investigation, as it possesses marked medicinal properties. The direction of experiment may be judged by reference to the Dispensatory. Use a tincture of the recently dried root, in doses of 30 to 60 drops.

CELASTRUS SCANDENS.
(FALSE BITTERSWEET.)

This belongs to the class alterative. It has no special action that I am aware of, though it might be studied with advantage.

CHELONE GLABRA.
(BALMONY.)

The Chelone exerts an influence on waste and nutrition, and deserves study. We would prepare a tincture from the recent leaves, by expression, in the proportion of ʒviij. to Alcohol, 76° Oj. Dose, ten to thirty drops.

CHIMAPHILLA UMBELLATA.
(PIPSISSEWA.)

The Chimaphilla has been used mostly in infusion or decoction: but for general use it may be prepared in the form of tincture, both of the *recent* and the dried leaves—though they will differ materially in strength and properties—the fresh leaves possessing a volatile principle which is lost in drying.

The Chimaphilla has been principally employed as a tonic diuretic, influencing the urinary apparatus in a similar manner to the Buchu and Uva-Ursi, though I think it preferable to either. It relieves irritation of the entire urinary tract, and improves the circulation and nutrition of these organs.

It also influences the processes of waste and nutrition, and possesses the properties termed alterative. In this respect it has not been thoroughly studied, though highly spoken of by some in the treatment of scrofula and secondary syphilis.

CHIONANTHUS VIRGINICA.
(FRINGE-TREE.)

This agent comes to us with the recommendation of Dr. I. J. M. Goss, of Georgia, who says:

"It possesses important alterative properties. As a catalytic, it has the most decided influence over the glandular system of any article I have tried. It pervades the whole system, combining with the materies morbi, and conveying it out of the system. I have used it in mercurial cachexy with the most happy success, in quite a number of instances. But the most important therapeutical property that it possesses, is its specific power over morbid conditions of the liver. I have tried it in hypertrophy of that organ, and with uniform success; and also in obstruction of the liver, in malarious districts, with like success. Some years ago I called the attention of the profession to its specific effects in jaundice, and gave several cases in proof of the fact. Since then I have used the Chionanthus in a great many cases of jaundice, and have never failed to remove it in but one single case, and that one I think was a case of obstruction of the gall ducts by calculi ; in that case, I tried all the reputed cholagogues, without success. It removes jaundice of years standing, in from eight to ten days. I have treated several persons that had been subject to jaundice, annually, in summer, for several years, and had been dosed with blue pill, calomel, and other articles, without any benefit, and I have not failed in a single instance, to remove the disease entirely. And when it is relieved with the Chionanthus, it does not return ; at least it has not, in any instance to my knowledge. It is as near a specific in jaundice, as quinine in periodicity. The mode in which I have used it is to make a tincture of the bark of the root in gin, say ʒij. to the quart of gin, and give ʒss. of this every three hours, or the fluid extract, and give from one to two drachms every three hours."

CHLOROFORM.

Chloroform by inhalation exerts a *specific* influence upon the cerebral center, arresting its power to receive impressions—a condition known as anæsthesia. If carried still farther, it influences the spinal center

in the same manner, and arrests automatic movement—respiration. This action is so well known,
that it is not worth while occupying our space
with it.

Administered by mouth, in small doses, it is a
cerebral stimulant; in large doses, it lessens consciousness, the effect being more like poisoning by
Alcohol, than the anæsthetic influence from its inhalation.

In small doses (gtts. x. to ʒj.) it is successfully
employed to arrest convulsions. The small doses
are safe, but it will not do to repeat it often in the
larger quantity named. It is also used to relieve
gastro-intestinal pains, especially in the form of
common colic.

In cases of *biliary calculus* it is used as a prophylactic, preventing the deposit of cholesterin, and
causing its solution when deposited. For this purpose it is used in doses of gtts. xx., three times a
day.

CHLORAL HYDRATE.

The introduction of this new remedy has been
attended with the same enthusiasm displayed in the
case of Bromide of Potassium. It is evidently good
for something, but what, has not yet been satisfac-
torily determined.

It is a *hypnotic*, and may be employed for this
purpose, where there is an enfeebled condition of the
brain, with impaired nutrition. It relieves pain,

when the nervous centers are suffering from impaired circulation and irritation, and may be advantageously employed in these cases.

It has been successfully employed in the treatment of *delirium tremens*, but in some cases it has failed. I have not used it for this purpose, but applying the above principles would conclude that it is a remedy only in those in which the nervous centers are suffering the *exhaustion* of over stimulation, and not in those in which there is irritation and determination of blood. These cases require opposite remedies, and if I am correct in the view I have taken of the action of Chloral, it will doubtless prove a very important remedy.

The remedy also suggests itself as one adapted to allay irritation and produce sleep in a majority of cases of puerperal mania. Dr. Playfair reports a case in which it was used with excellent success.

I am satisfied from its action that it will prove a boon to the *opium eater* who desires to break off the destructive habit. Whilst its influence upon the nerve centers is the same as stimulant doses of Opium, and will thus give present relief, it gives strength to the cerebral circulation, and will thus favor normal nutrition; then the dose can be lessened, and finally the remedy dispensed with.

To give the estimate in which the drug is now held, I quote from the *London Lancet:*

" This interesting drug has now been sufficiently tested by a large number of eminent practitioners to enable us to form a tolerably clear idea both of

its merits and its defects; and as we perceive t
(after the usual fashion in matters medical) there
going to be an epidemic rage for the new reme
it may be well to call the attention of the public
the principal features of its action which can
said to be fairly made out.

"In the first place, the term 'anæsthetic' shou
no longer be applied to chloral, for it has entir
failed to make good its claim to this reputatic
even the largest doses do but produce a heavy a
prolonged sleep, which is, however, essentially c
ferent from true anæsthesia. On the other hand,
a producer of sleep, Chloral is, in many respec
unrivaled; for though, like every other remedy
fails in a considerable number of cases, it does s
ceed in a very large number; in fact, it is infer
in certainty, as a hypnotic, to Opium alone. Mo
over, it is very greatly superior to Opium, a
almost every other drug, in the character of
sleep-producing action; there are no attenda
symptoms of cerebral oppression; the sleep, thou
often prolonged, is light and refreshing, and no t
pleasant after-symptoms are experienced. It is i
portant to observe, however, that this descripti
only applies to the use of moderate quantities, a
that not only unpleasant but highly danger
symptoms have been produced by doses which
regret to see are very commonly used. Very care
inquiry leads us to assert that it is both unnecessa
and dangerous to give larger doses than twenty
thirty grains, repeated once or twice if necessa

for hypnotic purposes. Doubtless it might happen that 100 consecutive patients might take much larger doses with impunity, but the 101st might present the alarming symptoms described by Dr. Reynolds, in a recent number of the *Practitioner*, as produced by a dose of fifty grains, and these symptoms might easily take a fatal turn.

"As a remedy for pain, Chloral holds a very varying place in the estimation of medical men, some rating it highly, and others thinking it almost worthless. Perhaps the safest estimate of its power over pain is that it only exerts an indirect influence by inducing a disposition to sleep, in which the pain is forgotten. Certainly it has entirely failed, in the hands of the present writer, to relieve severe pain of a pure neuralgic type. On the other hand, there is a good deal of evidence that it relieves suffering where the parts are very *tense*, and where mere arterial *throbbing* counts for much in the production of pain; thus it has been very favorably spoken of for its effects in gout. And this fact, if it be correct, corresponds with certain observations which have been made as to its action on the circulation. Both from sphygmographic experiments on healthy persons and on patients, and also from the details of the nearly fatal case reported by Dr. Reynolds, there is reason to think that Chloral exerts a contracting influence upon the arteries, powerful in proportion to the dose; and it may well be that arterial throbbing is checked by this kind of influence.

"On the whole, however, there can be little doubt

10

that the great function of Chloral is that of a hypnotic and calmer of general nervous irritability. In delirium tremens it is excellent: and it is probable that with two such weapons for choice as Bromide of Potassium and Chloral we shall be able almost entirely to dispense with the use of Opium, which is so uncertain and dangerous a remedy in that disease. In the state of sleeplessness which threatens the access of puerperal mania, Chloral is probably an unequaled remedy. In melancholia its action as a hypnotic appears to be powerfully and remarkably sure. In mania, also, it acts well enough as a hypnotic, though there seems some division of opinion as to whether it does permanent good. We may also state that in the irritable condition of aged persons who find it difficult to sleep for any length of time continuously, the use of a single dose of thirty grains of Chloral appears often to answer excellently well. The minor uses of the drug in relieving more trivial conditions of nervous irritation, and in alleviating painful spasmodic symptoms of various kinds, are probably considerable."

CINCHONA.—(*See Quinia.*)

CISTUS CANADENSIS.
(Rock-Rose.)

Preparation.—A tincture is prepared from the recent plant, in the proportion of ℥viij. to Alcohol 76° Oj. The dose is from ten to thirty drops.

The Cistus has a direct and positive influence on the processes of waste and nutrition, and hence possesses the properties known as *alterative*. It has been used with especial advantage in scrofula, and in chronic diseases dependent upon an enfeebled nutrition, or deposit of imperfectly formed plasma.

It is also reported to have a specific influence upon the intestinal canal, curing chronic diarrhœa and dysentery. It deserves a thorough investigation, which I trust some of our practitioners will give it.

CINNAMON.

Preparation.—We prepare a tincture from the oil, in the proportion of ʒj. to Alcohol 98° ℥viij. Dose five to thirty drops.

Cinnamon thus prepared exerts a direct influence upon the uterus, causing contraction of its muscular fibre, and arresting hemorrhage. To a limited extent, it exerts an influence on the entire circulatory system, checking hemorrhage from any part.

It is the most certain remedy we have for uterine hemorrhage, either during parturition or at the menstrual period. I have used it since I commenced practice, and have never failed to arrest post-partum hemorrhage with it, though I have had some very severe cases.

CLEMATIS VIRGINIANA.
(Virgin's Bower.)

This agent has not been studied, though it deserves investigation. Prepare a tincture from the recent leaves, in the proportion of ℥viij. to Alcohol 76° Oj., using pressure. Dose, gtts. v. to gtts. x. To determine its influence upon the nervous system and upon the secretions.

COFFEE, (Java or Rio.)

Take of the berries of Coffee, ground (not roasted) ℥viij., Alcohol, 76° Oj. Make a tincture by percolation. Dose gtts. ij. to gtts. x.

Coffee is a stimulant to the cerebral nervous system, and may be employed in many cases where there is atony, with disordered function. Were it not for the general use of coffee as a beverage, it would prove a valuable remedy; but when persons are habituated to its use, it exerts but little influence.

COLLINSONIA CANADENSIS.
(Stone Root.)

We employ an alcoholic fluid extract of the Collinsonia, representing the crude article ounce for ounce. As there are a great many imperfect preparations in the market, I would advise that it be procured from one of our own houses in this city.

Collinsonia is a specific in ministers' sore throat;

administered in the proportion of : ℞ Fluid Extract of Collinsonia, Simple Syrup, aa., half teaspoonful to a teaspoonful four times a day.

It proves beneficial in other cases of chronic laryngitis, in chronic bronchitis, and phthisis, allaying irritation, and checking cough.

It also exerts a favorable influence upon the digestive processes, improving the appetite, facilitating digestion, and acting as a general tonic.

It passes off through the kidneys, and exerts a tonic influence upon the entire extent of the urinary tract.

I have thought that its influence was specially exerted upon and through the *pneumogastric*, relieving irritation of, and giving strength to parts supplied from this source.

Collinsonia is a specific in the early stages of hemorrhoids, and will sometimes effect a cure in the advanced stages of the disease. In this case it is employed in small doses : ℞ Fluid Extract of Collinsonia, ʒj. ; Water, ʒiv. ; a teaspoonful four times a day.

I have given the therapeutics of Collinsonia thus briefly, that the points named might make the greater impression upon the reader. I regard it as one of the most direct and valuable agents of the Materia Medica, and one that will give satisfaction to whoever employs it.

COLCHICUM.

It is difficult to procure a reliable preparation of Colchicum, and we have been obliged to use the English wine of Colchicum. Our manufacturers in this city now prepare a fluid extract, representing ounce for ounce of the crude article. The medium dose is one drop; we do not desire a cathartic action.

Colchicum has long been used as a remedy for rheumatism and gout; and, though probably the best of the old Materia Medica, it failed of giving its best results, because used in poisonous doses. In acute and chronic rheumatism it should be employed in small doses, following or alternated with the sedatives. We only obtain its anti-rheumatic influence when the pulse and temperature are reduced to nearly a normal standard.

It is also beneficial in some cases of intestinal disturbance, especially when there are gaseous accumulations. Thus in colic from intestinal irritation, it may be employed in the proportion of gtts. xx. to water, ℥iv., a teaspoonful every two hours, with prospect of success.

It exerts an influence upon the skin, and may occasionally be employed with advantage in chronic disease of the surface.

COLOCYNTH.

Colocynth has been employed as a cathartic, but for this purpose it is harsh and uncertain, and may *well be* dispensed with.

I use it wholly as a remedy for *dysentery*. And for this purpose employ the alcoholic fluid extract, in small doses, usually gtts. v. to Water ℥iv. A teaspoonful every hour will give the best results.

It will also prove beneficial in some cases of colic, and in diarrhœa attended with tormina and tenesmus. I am satisfied that a thorough investigation of the remedy in small doses, will develop other important uses.

CYPRIPEDIUM PUBESCENS.
(LADY'S SLIPPER.)

Preparation.—Prepare a tincture from the recent dried root, in the proportion of ℥viij. to Alcohol 76° Oj. The dose will range from gtts. ij. to ℨj.

The Cypripedium is a nerve stimulant, improving the circulation and nutrition of the nerve centers. Hence it proves useful in sleeplessness, nervous irritability from atony, in neuralgia, delirium, and other disturbances from the same cause.

It is a feeble agent, and too much must not be expected from it. It is a stimulant, and will only be applicable in nervous atony.

Its best use will doubtless be found in children, to soothe irritation of the nervous system. I make the following prescription which is an admirable " Soothing Syrup."

℞ Tinct. of Cypripedium,
  Comp. Tinct. of Lavender, aa. ℨij.
  Tinct. of Lobelia, ℨj.
  Simple Syrup, ℥iss.   M.

CARBOLIC ACID.

We prepare Carbolic Acid for dispensing in general practice by adding ℥iv. of the crystals to ℥xvj. of Glycerine. In this form it is easily carried, and dispensed by adding the proper portion to water, so that the dose may be one teaspoonful.

Carbolic Acid exerts a specific influence in those cases in which, with a broad moist tongue, there is a cadaverous odor in the breath. It makes little difference what the name of the disease is—whether bilious or typhoid fever, cynanche, pneumonia, diarrhœa, dysentery, disease of the urinary apparatus, or whether the disease is acute or chronic. In these cases it is used in small doses as—℞ Solution of Carbolic Acid in Glycerine, gtts. x. to gtts. xxx.; Water, ℥iv.; a teaspoonful every hour.

We employ it with marked advantage in cases of irritable stomach, and to check nausea and vomiting, when the symptoms above named present. The faintest trace of the odor of putrescent meat will be an indication.

As far as my experience goes, it can not be used with advantage where the mouth is dry, or if the tongue is contracted, or elongated and pointed.

As a topical application, we employ Carbolic Acid when we need an antiseptic and a stimulant. Even here there must be the local symptoms, *fullness and relaxation* of tissues; whenever there is contraction, shrinking and dryness it will prove harmful. These rules hold good, whether as a dressing for wounds, for erysipelas, for burns, for a chancre, for a gargle, a vaginal injection, or for the treatment of a gonorrhœa or gleet.

It is an admirable dressing in many cases of cancer. Not so much as a curative remedy, as a palliative, and to arrest the rapid progress of the disease and destruction of tissue. It has proven especially valuable in the treatment of cancerous disease of the cervix uteri, in some cases arresting the progress of the disease for years. Even in these cases *fullness and relaxation of tissue, with putrescent odor*, is the indication for use.

The strength of the solution will vary in different cases. In some the full strength of the solution in Glycerine can be continually applied; in a few the full strength of the Acid, rendered fluid by heat; but in others it will require dilution with Glycerine. Use that strength that gives greatest ease, and leaves the parts in best condition. One of the principal objects is relief from pain, Carbolic Acid being a true anæsthetic in these cases, and the strength of the solution will be adapted to this use.

CUPRUM.

(COPPER.)

For some years I have prescribed Copper in the potent form of arsenic nickles, with most marked advantage in some cases of chronic disease. Even now I prefer to give Copper in this form, rather than as a medicine, but probably this is owing to

11

The cases where I have found it especially beneficial, were those in which with anæmia there was
not very great loss of flesh.   The surface would be
pallid, or sometimes tawny, the skin waxy, parts
usually colored with blood pale, with sometimes a
slight greenish tinge.   The tongue broad, pallid,
but usually clean; bowels torpid.   The pulse rather
full, but without sharpness of stroke.

It makes no difference what the disease is, if
these symptoms should present I would think of
Copper as a remedy.

Rademacher employed Copper in the treatment
of acute disease, and claimed that there were seasons
when the endemic constitution of disease demanded
it.   The symptoms calling for it were:—" The
color of the face was mostly palish-gray, dirty light
blue, seldom reddish, and only a few times, in
evening exacerbations, was it bright red and hot.
The palate was always red.   The sweats were moderate, sometimes clammy, and often smelt very
sour, and patients felt worse after them.   In most
cases there was a tendency to diarrhœa, or there
was more or less of diarrhœa present.   In pneumonia, patients complained of a sense of pressure
under the sternum and of weight in the chest;
though sometimes there would be no complaint,
until a sense of suffocation announced extensive infiltration of the lung."

Grauvogl accounts for the action of Copper in
this way:

" Science has already demonstrated that Copper,

in a finely divided state, absorbs immense quantities of ozone. It is also demonstrated that the ozone in the atmosphere is not found in the usual quantity in places, for example, which are affected by cholera, or, in which the atmospheric electricity is negative. Now Copper is one of the chief prophylactics against cholera, as we learn from workers in Copper, who remain free from cholera. Copper cures this disease in its first appearance, and in every case, so long as the consequences of the first stage have not set in, which naturally can no longer yield to the influence of Copper."

Speaking of water charged with a compound of cyanogen called iodosmone, he remarks:

" Moreover if one smells too often of this water, or drinks but even a small quantity thereof, he will experience in himself all the phenomena which precede cholera, followed by violent cholerine. The surest remedy to arrest, almost in a moment, this artificially produced state, is water impregnated with ozone. I convinced myself personally of the truth of this discovery. If we add to this the property of Copper in a finely divided state, of absorbing great quantities of oxygen, then the operation of Copper is explained according to a natural law; it operates inwardly, administered in a finely divided state as a function-remedy, as an ozone-bearer, since, circulating with the blood, it takes up more ozone from the inspired air than does the blood, and imparts it to the blood. Accordingly, all disease-forms, in which Copper is the

remedy, are to be referred to a lack of ozone, or
overplus of iodosmone in the blood, and these d
ease-forms naturally constitute as comprehensiv
group as the atmosphere forms a comprehens
condition of life."

CHELIDONIUM MAJUS.
(GREAT CELANDINE.)

Among the remedies used by the school of Ra
macher, Chelidonium held an important place.
was used for its *specific* influence upon the li
though its action undoubtedly extended to the
tire chylopoietic viscera. It has also been emplo
by French and German physicians to a limited
tent, and is a remedy valued by Grauvogl, tho
not much used by the mass of Homœopaths.

I have been experimenting with it for the
year, and its action has been so satisfactory in so
cases, that I am inclined to believe it will prov
valuable addition to our materia medica. I h
used the German tincture thus far, in the proj
tion of ʒj. to ʒij. to water ℥iv.; a teaspoonful ev
three or four hours. I propose, however, to ha
tincture prepared from our American plant as s
as possible, and test it; and I would recommen
any of my readers who know the plant—" G
Celandine, or Tetterwort "—to prepare a tinct
from the fresh herb and root, and test it.

I believe I can say that it acts on all the org
supplied from the solar plexus of nerves. In

olden time the liver was deemed the most important of these organs, and all diseases of the chylopoietic viscera were referred to it, hence the remedy was said to act specially upon the liver.

The cases in which it has seemed to me to exert the greatest influence, presnted the following symptoms: The tongue much enlarged, and somewhat pale; mucous membranes full and enfeebled; skin full and sallow, sometimes greenish; fullness in hypochondria; tumid abdomen; light colored feces; no abdominal pain; urine pale but cloudy, and of high specific gravity.

I have seen three cases of chronic disease presenting these symptoms, with the addition of œdema of the feet and legs, in two of which the influence of the Chelidonium was seemingly direct and curative. In one, it is associated with other means, and a sufficient time has not yet elapsed to determine the success, yet thus far it is beneficial. In one case of enlarged spleen, with confirmed dyspepsia, the influence was marked from the first, and in three weeks the patient concluded to dispense with medicine, and let nature complete the cure (because nature makes no charge for medicine.)

I do not wish to introduce the Chelidonium as a remedy that has been thoroughly studied, though it has a record in this direction of nearly one hundred years. But from my experience I think it is one that may be tested with advantage.

DATURA STRAMONIUM.
(JAMESTOWN WEED.)

Since the first edition of this work was published, I have been credibly informed that Stramonium is the principal agent in the "Opium Antidote," so extensively advertised during the last two years. A limited use of the agent in these cases goes to prove the truth of the information, and I would advise its trial, combined with a stomachic.

An ointment, prepared by boiling the fresh leaves in mutton tallow, furnishes an excellent local application for hemorrhoids, and ulceration of mucous surfaces.

DELPHINIUM STAPHISAGRIA.
(STAVESACRE.)

Preparation.—A tincture is prepared from the ground seed, (it having been pressed between *bibulous* paper to remove the fixed oil), in the proportion of ℥viij. to Alcohol 98° Oj.

The Tincture of Staphisagria has a specific action upon the reproductive organs of both male and female; but more marked in the first. It quiets irritation of the testes, and strengthens their function; it lessens irritation of the prostate and vesiculæ; arrests prostatorrhœa, and cures inflammation of these parts. It also exerts a marked influence upon the urethra, quieting irritation and ng mucous, or muco-purulent discharges; it influences the bladder and kidneys, but in less degree.

The action of Staphisagria upon the nervous system is peculiar. It exerts a favorable influence where there is depression of spirits and despondence, in cases of hypochondriasis and hysteria, especially when attended with moroseness, and violent outbursts of passion.

I employ it in the proportion of: ℞ Tincture of Staphisagria, ℨj ; Water, ℥iv. A teaspoonful every four hours.

The seed of the *Delphinum Consolida* or *Larkspur*, possesses similar medical properties, but is not so active ; a tincture may be prepared in the same way, and used in the same dose.

DIERVILLA CANADENSIS.
(Bush Honeysuckle.)

Preparation.—A tincture may be prepared from the recent leaves and twigs, ℥viij. to Alcohol 76° Oj. Dose gtts. x. to ℨj.

We have no positive knowledge with regard to this agent, though it is credited with active properties. It would be well to test its influence upon the urinary apparatus, and to increase waste and nutrition.

DIGITALIS PURPUREA.
(Foxglove.)

Prepare a tincture from the recent dried leaves in the proportion of ℥viij. to Alcohol 76° Oj. Dose, from a fraction of one drop to five drops.—℞ Tincture of Digitalis, gtts. x. to xx.; Water, ℥iv. A teaspoonful every one or two hours.

Digitalis may be employed for the general purposes of a sedative, to lessen the frequency of the pulse, and the temperature, in cases of fever and inflammation. It is somewhat analogous to Aconite, and exerts the best influence in atonic conditions. For these purposes, however, it must be used in small doses.

It is a powerful cardiac tonic when used in small doses, and may be employed in any case of heart disease where the organ is enfeebled. It not only gives the necessary stimulation for the present, but it gives a permanent improvement; doubtless through an improved nutrition.

It exerts an influence upon the capillary circulation, and may be employed with much certainty to arrest asthenic hemorrhages. It also influences the absorption of dropsical deposits, and increases secretion from the kidneys, probably in the same way.

There is no *cumulative* effect when Digitalis is used in small doses.

DIOSCOREA VILLOSA.
(WILD YAM.)

An infusion of the recent Dioscorea will undoubtedly give the best results. A tincture may be prepared from the recent root in the proportion of ℥viij. to Alcohol 76° Oj. Dose gtts. x. to ℥j.

The article that has been sold for Dioscorea by most of our druggists for the past ten years, and from which the Dioscorein has been prepared, is a species of *smilax*. A very good joke on Dioscorein! but unpleasant to those who have expected it to relieve pain in the bowels.

True Dioscorea, when recent, is a specific in bilious colic, when given in infusion, or even in tincture. In any case it allays gastro intestinal irritation, and favorably influences the vegetative processes. It is a feeble but certain diaphoretic, and allays irritation of the nervous system.

DROSERA ROTUNDIFOLIA.
(Sundew.)

We employ a tincture of the fresh plant prepared in Germany, using it in the proportion of: ℞ Tincture of Drosera, gtts. x. to ℥j.; Water, ℥iv. A teaspoonful every three or four hours.

I use the Drosera as a specific in the cough attending and following measles, especially where there is dryness of the respiratory mucous membranes. An experience of ten years with it, in a large number of cases, has given me great confidence in the remedy.

We also use it in cases of whooping cough, especially where there is dryness of the air-passages, and much irritation of the nervous system. Whilst it is not a remedy for all cases of whooping cough, it is a true specific in those to which it is ministered. I have often seen a serious case of the disease relieved in twenty-four hours, and an entire arrest of the cough in two weeks.

We may employ it in cases of chronic cough, with dryness of the air-passages and nervous irritation, with much advantage. It makes little difference whether it arises from bronchial irritation or inflammation or paralysis, if associated with irritation of the basilar portions of the brain, and pneumogastric.

EPIGÆA REPENS.
(Trailing Arbutus.)

This remedy deserves further and careful investigation. We wish to determine its influence upon the urinary apparatus, and the intestinal canal.

For this purpose a tincture of the fresh leaves may be prepared with dilute alcohol.

EPILOBIUM PALUSTRE.

For general use the infusion is the preferable form for administration; but we have a tincture prepared with dilute alcohol, employing pressure.

The Epilobium exerts a specific influence upon the intestinal mucous membrane, relieving irritation, and promoting normal function. Thus, it is employed in acute diarrhœa and dysentery, and in colic, with advantage. I have also prescribed it to quiet the irritation and check the diarrhœa in typhoid fever, with marked benefit.

It is especially valuable, however, in chronic

diarrhœa and dysentery; sometimes effecting cures where all other means had failed. Thus, I employed it extensively in the treatment of the chronic diarrhœa during the recent war, and with a success not to be obtained from other remedies. I do not pretend to account for its action, but its curative influence is well established.

ERECHTHITES HIERACIFOLIUS.
(FIREWEED.)

Preparation.—A tincture may be prepared from the recent plant, in the usual proportions, using alcohol of 76°. Dose from gtts. x. to ʒj.

We have here another remedy that requires study. It influences mucous tissue, especially of the bowels and lungs, and this will be the direction of the investigation.

ERIGERON CANADENSE.
(CANADA FLEABANE.)

We employ the Oil of Erigeron in practice, for the arrest of hemorrhage. For passive hemorrhage it is one of the most valuable remedies we have, and may be relied upon in hemorrhage from any organ or part. For this purpose the dose will be from five to ten drops on sugar, as often as may seem necessary.

The Erigeron influences the kidneys in a manner similar to Buchu. It may be employed in diabetes and albuminuria with advantage; also, in chronic

inflammation of the kidneys, bladder and urethra.
Latterly it has been recommended for gonorrhœa.

ERYNGIUM AQUATICUM.
(Water Eryngo.)

The Eryngium may be employed in infusion, or
in the form of a tincture of the recent dried root,
℥viij. to proof spirit, Oj.   Dose, gtts. x. to gtts. xx.

The Eryngium exerts a specific influence upon
the bladder and urethra, relieving irritation.   It is
one of the most certain remedies that can be employed in dysuria from irritation, and in spasmodic
stricture; continued, it proves curative in these
cases.

It has been employed for other purposes, and we
find it highly recommended.   It undoubtedly deserves a thorough investigation.

EUONYMUS ATROPURPUREUS.
(Wahoo.)

Preparation.—Prepare a tincture from the bark of
the recent root, in the proportion of ℥viij. to Alcohol 76° Oj.   Dose, gtts. x. to ℥j.

The Euonymus stimulates the nutritive processes,
and in some cases improves digestion.   Usually,
however, it will need to be combined with a pure
bitter, as the hydrastis, to get its full action in this
direction.

It exerts a marked influence in malarial diseases,
and deserves the name of an antiperiodic, though it

is much feebler than Quinine. It may, however, be used in these cases with marked advantage, after the fever has been once broken.

EUPATORIUM AROMATICUM.
(WHITE SNAKEROOT.)

Preparation.—Prepare a tincture from the recent dried root, in the proportion of ʒviij. to Alcohol 76° Oj. Dose, gtts. x. to ʒj.

This variety of the Eupatorium exerts a marked influence upon the brain, relieving irritation and promoting normal action. It is also diaphoretic, and probably influences, to a slight degree, all of the functions governed by the sympathetic. It will repay careful investigation.

EUPATORIUM TEUCRIFOLIUM.
(WILD HOARHOUND.)

Preparation.—Prepare a tincture from the recent plant, using dilute alcohol. The dose will vary from one drop to one drachm.

In small doses it stimulates all the functions controlled by the sympathetic nervous system; improving digestion, blood making, and stimulates waste and excretion. It may be combined with a simple bitter tonic, or preparation of iron, or the hypophosphites, for its restorative influence, or with the vegetable alteratives for its other use.

In large doses it is a powerful diaphoretic.

EUPATORIUM PURPUREUM.
(QUEEN OF THE MEADOW.)

Preparation.—Prepare a tincture from the recent root, in the proportion of ℥viij. to Alcohol 98° Oj. Dose, gtts. x. to f℥ss.

Its principal influence is upon the kidneys, and it may be employed whenever an increased volume of urine is desirable.

It has been mostly employed in the treatment of dropsy, with reported success.

Its influence upon the urinary organs may doubtless be made valuable, but it requires further study.

EUPATORIUM PERFOLIATUM.
(BONESET.)

Preparation.—Prepare a tincture from the recently dried herb in the proportion of ℥viij. to proof spirit Oj. Dose from gtts. v. to ℥j.

The Eupatorium increases functional activity of the skin, and to a less extent, secretion from the kidneys. It also influences the circulation, to a slight extent, and does well combined with the sedatives.

In quite small doses it stimulates the sympathetic nervous system, and improves all the vegetative functions. It is not an active remedy, and too much must not be expected from it; yet, in many cases, it may well supplant costly foreign drugs.

EUPHORBIA COROLLATA.—E. IPECACUANHA.
(Bowman's Root—Wild Ipecac.)

Preparation.—Prepare a tincture of the first from the bark of the root, of the second, from the root, (dried), ℥viij. to Alcohol 76° Oj.   Dose, gtts. j. to x.

These remedies have not been sufficiently studied; yet, possessing active properties, they are likely to prove valuable.   The Euphorbia Corollata exercises a direct influence upon the mucous surfaces, relieving irritation, and promoting functional activity. This is noticed more especially in the digestive tract.   In quite small doses it improves digestion, both stomachic and intestinal, tends to overcome constipation and irregularity.

It may be employed with advantage in some forms of diarrhœa and dysentery, using it in the place of Ipecac.   To arrest inflammatory action in the intestinal canal, seems to be its specific use.

FERRUM.
(Iron.)

We employ three preparations of Iron—Metallic Iron in powder, the Tincture of Chloride of Iron, and the Tincture of Acetate of Iron.   The first is Iron by Hydrogen, or Quevenne's; a good article may be known by its iron-gray color and its effervescing with acids; the spurious is black, and effervesces but slighly.   The Tincture of Chloride of Iron should be ordered of a reliable manufacturer.   *It will* be a clear, deep-colored tincture,

without a trace of yellowness or deposit at the
bottom of the bottle.

We employ Iron as a restorative. It is a component part of the red corpuscles, and experience has
shown that its administration stimulates the formation of these bodies. In proportion as the red corpuscles are increased, blood-making becomes more
active and nutrition is improved. It thus becomes
a very important remedy in cases of anæmia, with
impaired nutrition.

As a restorative, it is better to administer the
necessary quantity of Iron with the food. Experiment has demonstrated that at other times it is appropriated slowly or not at all. It does not require
a very large amount to accomplish the object, for
Iron exists in small quantity in the body. The dose
of Metallic Iron need never be more than five grains,
often not more than one; whilst of the Tincture,
the dose will be from five to twenty drops.

In the selection of the preparation I would be
guided by the appearance of the mucous membrane.
If it is deep-red, use the Tincture of Chloride, if
pallid, Metallic Iron.

We also employ Iron as a specific against certain
zymotic poisons. The reader has probably employed
The Tincture of Chloride in erysipelas, and many
regard it as a true specific in the disease, rarely
making any other prescription. I think we may
say, that in all cases of erysipelas presenting the
deep-red discoloration of mucous membranes, with
the same deep color of the local disease, the Tinc-

ture may be prescribed with great confidence. But my experience with the disease has shown me that where the mucous membranes are pallid, the coating of the tongue white and pasty, the Sulphite of Soda is the best remedy. In these cases Quevenne's Iron might be tested.

Rademacher claimed that Iron was specific to one of his three *epidemic constitutions*. This was characterized by pallor of the skin, moderate heat, with a small, thin or soft, empty pulse. His description, so far as I have seen it in translation, is so meager that we can hardly determine the condition in which he valued it so highly, even treating all the cases of pneumonia in a season with Iron alone.

The preparation of Iron employed by the school of Rademacher was a Tincture of the Acetate, prepared by the following formula:

"Take of pure Sulphate of Iron two ounces and seven drachms; of the pure Acetate of Lead three ounces; triturate them together in an Iron mortar so long as may be needed to reduce them to a soft conformable mass; then put the mass in an iron vessel with six ounces of distilled water and twelve ounces of diluted Acetic Acid; heat the mixture until it boils. After it has become cold, add six ounces of pure Alcohol.

"The mixture is then to be put in a glass vessel with a ground stopper for at least six months—to be shaken daily—when it will acquire a high red color; then it is to be filtered through paper.

"By this long process the Tincture will have a
12

mild, pleasant taste, and a smell similar to Malaga Wine, more noticeable on the addition of Gum Arabic to the mixture. The older the mixture is the pleasanter the smell and taste, and hence it is desirable to make it in large quantities."

A simpler formula than the above is the one of the Dublin Pharmacopœia, on page 1253 King's Dispensatory.

It is prescribed in doses of gtts. v. to ℥j; and will be found an excellent preparation where Iron is indicated, and we do not wish the Muriatic Acid.

Recent investigation has shown that the solid blue coloration of tongue is an indication for small doses of Iron in any disease. For this I would prescribe Tinct. Acetate of Iron, ℥ij.; Water, or Syrup, ℥iv.; a teaspoonful every three or four hours.

The majority of our readers are well acquainted with the use of Tincture of Muriate of Iron in erysipelas, and have administered it in this disease with a certainty that they rarely feel with regard to other remedies. I don't think any one, even the most skeptic with regard to specific medication, will question the specific action of this remedy in many cases of this disease. And as it is such a well known example, we will use it to illustrate certain facts in therapeutics.

The first proposition I will make is, that it is not specific to all cases of erysipelas. Whilst in some, embracing some of the severest, it is the only remedy needed, in others you might quite as well give water, other than the iron proves a topical irritant.

We ask the question, then, in what condition of this disease is it specific, and what are the symptoms indicating its use? Or, in what conditions is it contra-indicated, and what are the evidences that show this?

It is easier to pick out the case where other treatment will be preferable, and where we would not use the iron. In any case of erysipelas, with a full bounding, or full hard pulse, and bright redness of the local disease, I would always prefer Veratrum as an internal and a topical remedy. Indeed, nothing is more certain than Veratrum in these cases. Take again the case presenting the broad, pallid tongue, with moist, pasty coat, and I would very certainly prefer Sulphite of Soda; or if it was a moist, dirty tongue, without so much pallor, Sulphurous Acid.

Is it possible to point out the indications for Iron? I think it will be if we examine those cases specially in which Iron is the remedy. One of the most pronounced symptoms that I have noticed is a peculiar solid blue color of mucous membranes, sometimes deepening into purple when there is a determination. The same change in color may sometimes be noticed in the local disease. In several cases of simple erysipelas, I have been tempted to prescribe Tincture of Muriate of Iron from this appearance, and with good results. I hope our readers will study this point carefully and see if I am correct. If not, find a certain indication for its use.

Now for the argument. Take a case of erysipelas of the severest type, in which Iron is the remedy—what are the results of its administration *alone?* The pulse is 120 to 130, small and hard; within forty-eight hours it comes down to 80, and is soft and open. The temperature is probably 106°; in forty-eight hours it comes down to 100°. The skin is dry and harsh, the urine scanty and high colored, the bowels constipated; in forty-eight hours the skin is soft and moist, the urine free, the bowels act without medicine. The nervous system is in a state of extreme irritation, possibly the patient is delirious; in forty-eight hours the patient is conscious and the suffering relieved. Here we have the most marked effect of a *sedative, diaphoretic, diuretic, laxative, and cerebro-spinant,* and yet we have given but the one remedy, Tincture of Muriate of Iron. Now I ask the question, why these results?

You answer, because the Iron specifically antagonized the blood-poison. Yet Tincture of Muriate of Iron is not regarded as an antiseptic, and we have a number of cases of erysipelas, in which Iron does not antagonize the blood poison.

How is this? Is it not well worth thinking of? And if Tincture of Muriate of Iron thus becomes a specific to a certain form of grave zymotic disease, may we not hope to find other remedies of a similar character?

I present the subject in this form, that we may think of it, and hope at some future time to give a rational explanation of some of these facts in therapeutics.

FRASERA CAROLINENSIS.
(AMERICAN COLUMBO.)

Preparation.—Prepare a tincture from the fresh root, in the proportion of ℥viij. to Alcohol 98° Oj. Dose, gtts. j. to v.

This remedy has been but little used, and that little has been of the dried root as a tonic. The recent root possesses quite active properties, and is likely to repay investigation. It is stimulant to the circulation, and will doubtless exert the same influence upon all the vegetative functions. Will some one give it a thorough study and report?

FUCUS HELMINTHOCORTON.
(CORSICAN MOSS.)

Prepare a Tincture in the usual manner, using dilute Alcohol. Dose from gtts. v. to ℥ss.

We wish to determine its influence upon the functions of waste and nutrition, and especially in cases of degenerations and growths. It has had some reputation in the treatment of benign and malignant growths. It exerts a direct influence upon the intestinal canal, and this may suggest the course of experiment.

FRAXINUS SAMBUCIFOLIA—F. ACUMINATA.
(ASH.)

Preparation.—Prepare a tincture from the recent bark, in the proportion of ℥viij. to Alcohol 76° Oj. Dose from gtts. ij. to f℥ss.

Both the *black* and *white* ash deserve study. The first, for its influence in skin diseases, especially of an herpetic character, and ~~as a~~ general alterative. The second, to improve secretion, and for its influence upon the chylopoietic viscera.

GALIUM APARINE.
(CLEAVERS.)

Galium is most frequently employed in infusion, especially for its influence upon the urinary apparatus. A tincture may be prepared from the recent herb by expression, using only sufficient alcohol for preservation.

The first use of Galium is to relieve irritation of the urinary apparatus, and increase the amount of urine. For this purpose it will be found one of our best remedies. In dysuria and painful micturition, it will frequently give prompt relief.

It has recently been employed in *cancer*, used locally and internally. A case of *hard nodulated tumor* of the tongue, apparently cancerous, is reported in the British Medical Journal, as having been cured with it. Whether it was cancerous or not, it suggests a line of experiment which may develop an important use of the remedy.

GAULTHERIA PROCUMBENS.
(WINTERGREEN.)

Preparation.—Prepare a tincture from the fresh plant, in the proportion of ℥viij. to Alcohol 98° Oj. Dose from gtts. ij. to gtts. x.

In this form and in these doses, the Gaultheria exerts a special influence upon the bladder, prostate and urethra, allaying irritation and inflammation. It may also be employed in dysuria. Probably one of its most important uses is, as an anaphrodisiac, exerting a direct and quite certain influence upon the reproductive organs of both male and female. For this purpose it is employed in some cases of spermatorrhœa. It will not do, however, to mistake the case, and use it where the venereal function is already impaired.

GELSEMINUM SEMPERVIRENS.
(YELLOW JESSAMINE.)

The commercial tincture has been so variable in strength that much harm has resulted from its use. In some cases the harm has been direct from over doses, in others, indirect from depending upon a feeble or worthless remedy. Before the war, we had a very crude tincture prepared from the green root, with proof spirits (whisky?), containing about as much of the medicinal properties as could be held by such spirit. During the war, there being difficulty in obtaining a supply of the root, and greater difficulty in having it shipped green, the tincture in the market gradually deteriorated until it was worthless. Even yet it has not regained its medicinal properties with many *druggers*.

We have thought that a good tincture could only be made from the fresh root. But some who have employed the dried root (not old), claim that it makes fully as reliable a tincture. Dr. Locke, of Newport, prepares his tincture from the dried root, and claims that it is more reliable than any he can buy.

It is not worth while to give a formula for the preparation of a tincture, as it will be purchased by a great majority of our readers. That which bears the label of "Specific Medicine" will be found very strong. Dose from gtts. j. to gtts. vj.

Gelseminum exerts a specific influence upon the brain, and to a less extent upon the spinal center and sympathetic. It relieves irritation and determination of blood, and the disordered innervation that flows from it. Probably there is no remedy in the Materia Medica that is more direct and certain in its action. Given, a case of irritation and determination of blood to the brain, marked by flushed face, bright eyes, contracted pupils, restlessness and irritability, we prescribe Gelseminum with certainty. This being a common complication in diseases of childhood, it is especially the child's remedy.

Acting in this direction, it lessens the frequency of the heart's action, and removes obstruction to the free flow of blood—a sedative. It also increases secretion in the same way.

I do not think the Gelseminum exerts any important influence, other than through this action upon the nervous system. But, as will be observed, this is a very important action.

It is contra-indicated where the circulation is feeble, and there is tendency to congestion. Especially if there is a feeble circulation in the nerve centres. We never give it if the eyes are dull, pupils dilated, and the countenance expressionless. In such cases, it may prove fatal in quite moderate doses. A number of these cases are on record, three or four in which death was produced by as small a dose as gtts. xxx. of a common tincture.

It has one other specific action, which is worthy of attention. It is the remedy in dysuria from stricture, and will rarely fail in enabling the patient to pass urine in from four to eight hours.

GENTIANA LUTEA.
(GENTIAN.)

Gentian is an excellent stomachic bitter, and resembles, in its medicinal action, our Hydrastis. I do not think, however, it has the same kindly influence in irritable conditions of the stomach.

A very fine preparation may be made by taking two parts of Gentian, and one part of Podophyllin, and making a tincture by percolation, using alcohol. It is one of the most efficient remedies I have ever used in atony of the stomach and bowels, with feeble or slow digestion.

GERANIUM MACULATUM.
(CRANESBILL.)

The Geranium is an astringent from the presence of Tannic and Gallic Acids in large quantity; and hence will possess the medicinal properties of these. It is claimed, however, to possess other properties, acting more kindly, and giving tone to mucous membranes. Whilst I believe the remedy has been over-rated, I am confident that experiment will develop some special use.

It may be employed in infusion with good results, especially when a topical action on the stomach and bowels is wanted, or in chronic cases when we desire the action of Gallic Acid. For general use I would suggest a tincture by percolation, using Alcohol of 80°. The Geranin, though not entirely worthless, is a feeble and costly medicine.

GERARDIA PEDICULARIA.

Will some of our Southern physicians give this remedy a trial and report. For experiment, make a tincture by percolation, ℥viij. to the Oj., using dilute Alcohol. Test it as a sedative, a diaphoretic, and an antiseptic.

GILLENIA TRIFOLIATA—G. STIPULACEA.
(INDIAN PHYSIC.)

Preparation.—Prepare a tincture from the root, in the proportion of ℥viij. to proof spirit, Oj. Dose from gtts. v. to ℥j.

These indigenous remedies possess marked medicinal properties, yet they have been so little used of late years that most physicians know nothing about them.

They deserve careful study. First, to determine their relation to Ipecac, and whether they will replace it in practice. The direction of the experiments may be seen by reference to this agent. We also wish to determine their influence upon the functions of digestion and secretion

GLYCERINE.

Glycerine is principally employed in medicine for its topical action. It is slightly stimulant to both skin and mucous membrane, and shields the skin from the action of the air. In many cases of simple cutaneous irritation, it will prove curative alone. In others, it will prove a good vehicle for the application of other remedies. In some cases of dyspepsia, Glycerine is a true remedy, allaying irritation, and giving gentle stimulation.

Glycerine is an admirable solvent, and may be used as a basis for many preparations, both for local use, and internal administration.

Notwithstanding the opposition, I still prefer the cheap Glycerine, manufactured in this city, to the higher priced Eastern and Foreign article. An extended use of Gordon's No. 1 Perfumer's Glycerine, has proved to me that it is the most bland of any article in the market. The slight odor is not as objectionable as the irritant properties developed by repeated distillation.

GNAPHALIUM POLYCEPHALUM.
(White Balsam.)

Preparation.—Prepare a tincture from the leaves, using Alcohol of 30°. Dose gtts. v. to 3ss.

This agent has been but little used, yet we think it worthy of investigation. The line of experiment will be, to determine its influence upon the urinary and reproductive organs—in acute and chronic ulcerations—and its action on the digestive apparatus.

GOSSYPIUM HERBACEUM.
(Cotton.)

Some years since the cotton-root was in considerable demand as an abortive. It was claimed that the Negro women of the South made common use of it, and that it was so certain and safe that they could rid themselves of the product of conception whenever they wished, and without impairment of health. It was singular what a demand sprung up for cotton-root bark; but fortunately for the unborn it had no influence on the gravid uterus.

Still the reports from the South seemed well authenticated, that, at least in some cases, it was abortive, and was a very certain emmenagogue, and a stimulant diuretic. It is only another example of a fact I have insisted on, that many plants possessing medicinal properties when fresh, lose them when dried, and especially when gathered at the wrong season and kept in stock.

If some of our manufacturers will get the bark of the cotton-root before the boll opens, and will prepare a tincture from it whilst fresh, we will probably find it possessing marked medicinal properties.

GUAIACUM OFFICINALE.

We prepare a tincture by percolation from the wood, in the proportion of ℥viij. to Alcohol 76° Oj. Dose, from ten to thirty drops.

The tincture thus prepared may be occasionally used with advantage in the latter stages of acute, and in chronic rheumatism. It may also be associated with the vegetable alteratives in the treatment of some chronic diseases, where stimulation of the skin is required. Occasionally it will prove useful in functional diseases of the uterine organs, especially in amenorrhœa.

GYMNOCLADUS CANADENSIS.
(AMERICAN COFFEE TREE.)

This agent has been but little used in medicine, yet if we are to judge from its common use as a *fly poison*, it possesses active properties that may be made available. For experiment, a tincture may be made of the bark, beans, or pulp of the seed-pod; the last being regarded as the most active.

Dr. Herring concluded from his experiments that it might be given with benefit in cases of "cough accompanied or followed by tonsilitis; in erysipelas of the face; in scarlet fever; in so-called hives; in typhoid fever; remittent or intermittent epidemic fever, with a typhoid character, etc."

The dose would be small. Of a tincture of ℥iv. of the pulp to the Oj.; gtts. x. to Water, ℥iv.; a teaspoonful every three hours would be sufficient.

HAMAMELIS VIRGINICA.
(WITCH-HAZEL.)

I prefer a distilled extract of the fresh leaves to any other preparation. That known to the trade as "Pond's Extract" is employed by most physicians who make use of the remedy. The ordinary fluid extract may be used as a topical application, as a gargle for the throat, and for the general purposes of an astringent.

Where the Witch Hazel can be readily obtained, I would advise that the leaves be gathered in June or July, and if no apparatus for distilling is at hand, that they be packed in a percolator, and a tincture prepared with a very weak spirit, say 30°.

I might say in this connection, that when I specify the strength of Alcohol by degrees, I have no reference to an imaginary standard of proof, but the figures represent the number of parts in one hundred.

The Hamamelis has a specific action upon the venous system, giving strength to it, and facilitating the passage of venous blood. It may, therefore, be employed with advantage in any case where a part is enfeebled, and there is a sluggish circulation. Thus we use it in cases of catarrh and ozœna; chronic pharyngitis, disease of the tonsils, pillars of the fauces, vellum and uvula, and in chronic laryngitis. The indications for its employment are, thickening of mucous membranes, with enfeebled circulation, and increased secretion, either mucous or muco-purulent.

It is especially a valuable remedy in the treatment of hemorrhoids, sometimes effecting a cure in old and very stubborn cases without the use of other remedies. Usually, however, I use the solution of the Persulphate of Iron as a local application.

It is also a very useful remedy in the treatment of diseases of the uterus and vagina. Given, a case with the conditions named, thickening, with relaxation, enfeebled circulation, and increased mucous, or muco-purulent secretion, and its action is very positive.

We employ it also in the treatment of various lesions of the lower extremities, both as a local application and an internal remedy, and many times with excellent results.

It is an excellent dressing for erysipelas, and for burns, giving that slight stimulation that seems to be required in these cases.

I need not name other cases, as the indications for its use first given, will suggest its application. I value the remedy very highly, and feel confident that a trial in the cases named will bring it into general use.

HEDEOMA PULEGIOIDES.
(PENNYROYAL.)

This is a much neglected article, probably be-cause it is so common. I regard it as one of the most valuable stimulant diaphoretics; very kindly received by the stomach, and quite certain in its action. As a remedy for colds it will prove very useful. To two ounces of the tincture add gtts. x. of Tincture of Veratrum, or ʒss. of Tincture of Ipecac, and give it in teaspoonful doses every one or two hours.

It is an admirable remedy for amenorrhœa from cold; the safest and most certain we have, I think. It may be given in doses of a teaspoonful every hour or two hours, or two or three times in the evening, with the hot foot bath.

Prepare your own tincture in this way: In July, gather a sufficient quantity of the herb, stem it, and at once pack the leaves in a percolator. Then add dilute Alcohol, or even common whisky, in the pro-portion of Oj. to each ʒviij. Let it stand twenty-four hours, and then draw off, putting on water until the tincture measures Oj. to each ʒviij.

HYPERICUM PERFOLIATUM.
(ST. JOHN'S WORT.)

Preparation.—We prepare a tincture from the fresh herb, ʒviij. to Oj., with alcohol of 50 per cent. The dose is small: of gtts. x. to gtts. xxx. to water ʒiv.; a teaspoonful every one or two hours.

According to our Homœpathic friends, the special

symptom indicating its use is, "sensation in the forehead as if touched by an ice-cold hand, in the afternoon, after which a spasmodic contraction in right eye." We would be glad to have the remedy thoroughly tested in diseases of the urinary apparatus, and in nervous affections with depression. Will some of our readers try it and report.

HELLEBORUS NIGER.
(BLACK HELLEBORE.)

Preparation.—A tincture is prepared in the usual way, using Alcohol of 76°. Dose gtts. ss. to gtts. x.

The black Hellebore is but little used, as in the dose recommended in the books it is an irritant poison. In small doses it is a stimulant to the spinal and sympathetic nervous systems, and it is probable that for this purpose it may be employed advantageously. I have used it with advantage in sterility of the female, and to increase virility in the male.

HELONIAS DIOICA.
(UNICORN ROOT.

True Helonias undoubtedly exerts a marked influence upon the reproductive organs of the female, but as it is so frequently supplied from the Aletris, but little dependence can be placed upon it.

It exerts the general influence of a tonic, and a special tonic action upon the uterine and urinary organs. It is possible that if we can obtain a reliable preparation, it will be found superior to other remedies *for these* purposes. One of the special in-

dications for its use is in the mental depression and
irritability that attends many of these affections. I
am of the impression that, in many cases, the relief
of this cerebral disturbance is its most important
action.

HEPATICA AMERICANA.
(LIVERLEAF).

Preparation.—Prepare a tincture from the fresh
leaves, using proof spirit. Dose gtts. v. to ʒss.

The Hepatica exerts a slightly stimulant and
tonic influence upon the stomach and small intestines, relieving irritation and promoting functional
activity. Thus it may be employed in atonic conditions of these and associate viscera with advantage.
Culpepper wrote, " It is a singular good herb for
all diseases of the liver, both to cool and cleanse it,
and is serviceable in yellow jaundice. It is a singular remedy to stay the spreading of tetters, ring-
worms, and other fretting and running sores."

It exerts an influence upon all mucous surfaces.
Probably its best action is upon the bronchial
mucous membrane, when enfeebled from irritation
or inflammation, attended with profuse secretion.
In these cases it may sometimes be given with great
benefit.

HERACLEUM LANATUM.
(MASTERWORT.)

This remedy has been but little used, but it might
repay careful study. It has been employed as an
antispasmodic, and we would judge that it was a

spinal stimulant. For experiment a tincture should be prepared from the green root.

The *Wild Parsnip* (Pastinaca Sativa) might also be tested. In poisonous doses, it produces great excitation of the nervous system, sometimes with convulsions, followed by coma and difficult respiration. This would suggest its use as a cerebro-spinal stimulant. Of course it would be used in *small* doses.

HYDRANGEA ARBORESCENS.
(Seven Barks.)

Preparation.—Prepare a tincture from the fresh or recently dried root, ℥viij. to the Oj., using Alcohol of 76°. Dose, gtts. x. to ℥ss.

This is a valuable remedy in diseases of the urinary apparatus. It gives tone to the kidneys, improving their functional activity, and thus tends to arrest the formation of urinary deposits and calculi. We do not believe, as Dr. J. W. Butler stated, that it will cure stone in the bladder, though it may prove prophylactic. It relieves irritation of the bladder and urethra, and hence proves serviceable in cases of gravel. It also exerts an influence upon the respiratory mucous tract, relieving bronchial irritation.

HYDRASTIS CANADENSIS.
Golden Seal.)

I will give the Hydrastis a brief notice, as it is in such general use for all the purposes of a tonic, that my readers know as much about it as I do. It improves the appetite and facilitates digestion; but beyond this it relieves gastro-intestinal irritation.

Its topical action, wherever applied, is that of a tonic, strengthening the circulation and nutrition. It is in common use for these purposes in diseases of the skin, diseases of the eyes, and diseases of mucous surfaces.

As a stomachic and tonic, I like the action of the finely powdered root, as well as the more costly preparations. Indeed, in most cases, I would prefer this, in equal quantity, to the Hydrastine.

A tincture made with Alcohol of 80° will be found a good preparation. It is more convenient for carrying, and added to water, gives a pleasant stomachic. A very good prescription would be: ℞ Tincture of Hydrastis, ℥ij.; Tincture of Nux Vomica, gtts. xx.; Water, ℥iv. A teaspoonful every three or four hours.

The *Sulphate of Hydrastia* is (when properly made) soluble in water in the proportion of four grains to the ounce. It makes a valuable collyrium in chronic conjunctivitis, or the latter stages of the acute. It is also an admirable injection in the second stages of gonorrhœa, and in gleet.

HYOSCYAMUS NIGER.
(HENBANE.)

Preparation.—We prepare a tincture from the recent dried leaves in the proportion of ℥viij. to Alcohol 76° Oj. Dose from gtts. ss. to gtts. v.

In medicinal doses, the Hyoscyamus is a stimulant to the cerebro-spinal centers, and may be employed whenever such action is desirable. It is from this that it has its sleep-producing properties, as well as the relief of pain. With some persons the tolerance for Hyosciamus is very great, and even drachm doses exert this stimulant influence.

It exerts a similar influence upon the vegetative system, in a slight degree favoring every process that is performed under its influence. It is not only stimulant, but it allays irritation. Thus, in some cases, when a frequent pulse is dependent upon irritation and debility of the cardiac nerves, it exerts the influence of the special sedatives. It never arrests secretion, but, as before remarked, it favors it. Thus small doses of Podophyllin, combined with Hyoscyamus, is not only less irritant, but more effectual. So we find in irritable states of the digestive apparatus, the addition of a small portion of Hyoscyamus to the bitter tonics improves their action.

Because Hyoscyamus is poisonous, it is no reason why it should be an active remedy. Poisoning and curing are too different things. Whilst it will be found a valuable curative agent, and quite direct in its action, its influence is rather feeble than otherwise, and too much must not be expected from it. The difference between a poison and a medicine, in this case, is a matter of dose alone, and in this respect it differs from some other medicines.

INULA HELENIUM.
(ELECAMPANE.)

Preparation.—Prepare a tincture from the fresh root, in the proportion of ℥viij. to Alcohol 50° Oj.

Elecampane is a feeble stimulant and tonic, but may sometimes be used for these properties with advantage. It not only exerts this influence upon the digestive tract, but also upon the skin, and is sometimes beneficial in chronic cutaneous diseases.

Its principal use, however, is in bronchial disease, with increased secretion. It may be used also in combination with Stillingia. Its action is slow, and it needs to be continued for some time to experience its benefits.

IODINE.

Iodine, in all its forms, increases retrograde metamorphosis, and, in some degree, stimulates excretion. We have no reason to believe that it stimulates blood-making or nutrition, other than as it facilitates the removal of worn-out tissues.

In quite small doses Iodine stimulates the sexual organs, and increases their power. For this purpose we may use it in the proportion of: ℞ Tincture of Iodine, gtts. xx.; Simple Syrup, ℥iv.; a teaspoonful four times a day.

Iodide of Potassium is doubtless its most active form as a resolvent and a stimulant of waste. There is great difference of opinion with regard to the proper dose; some think it best in doses of one to

five grains; others in doses of grs. **xx.** to **xl.** three
or four times a day. Of course our choice of dose
will depend upon the strength of the patient, the
character of the disease, and the rapidity of action
desired. As a remedy, it is greatly over-estimated.

The *Iodide of Sodium* has been but little used and
is obtained with difficulty in the market. I believe
that it is a better preparation than Iodide of Potassium, especially where there is asthenia and a feeble
circulation. The Iodide of Sodium may be employed with especial advantage in those cases that
present a pallid tongue and mucous membranes.

The *Iodide of Ammonium* should be selected when
stimulation of the nervous system is desirable.
Like the others, it increases waste, but it also improves nutrition, and does not impair digestion.
In secondary syphilis of an asthenic type, with nervous symptoms, this salt will be found an important remedy.

I would call especial attention to its action in
certain forms of chronic headache, depending upon
an enfeebled circulation and mal-nutrition. In
some of these cases it gives prompt relief, and effects
a permanent cure.

We prepare an Iodide of Ammonium for local
use as follows: ℞ Tincture of Iodine (strong),
Aqua Ammonia (strong), aa., put in a bottle and
allow it to stand until colorless. Its influence is
much better than the Tincture of Iodine alone; it
is less irritant and does not discolor the skin. It is
a favorite preparation with me in the treatment of

boils, local inflammations, buboes, etc., in the early stage, when we may expect resolution.

Iodide of Starch is an excellent preparation, affording the best means of giving Iodine without gastric irritation. It may be readily prepared in the office as follows : Triturate twenty-four grains of Iodine with a little water in a mortar, adding gradually an ounce of finely powdered starch, continuing the trituration until it assumes a uniform blue color. It is then dried with gentle heat, and kept in a well stopped bottle. The dose will vary from five grains to a teaspoonful, given in gruel.

IPECACUANHA.
(IPECAC.)

Preparation.—Prepare a tincture from the root (a good article) ℥viij. to Alcohol 76° Oj. Dose from the fraction of a drop to gtts. v.

Ipecacuanha exerts a specific influence upon mucous membranes, relieving irritation, and arresting the inflammatory process. It also stimulates a better circulation and innervation, increases nutrition, and thus favors functional activity.

We employ it as a specific in most cases of cholera infantum. It allays irritation of the stomach, gradually checks the frequency of the discharges from the bowels, and restores tone and functional activity. In a large experience in the treatment of this disease, we have found nothing to equal it. It is usually prescribed in the following proportions: ℞

Tincture of Ipecac, gtts. v. to gtts. xxx.; Water, ʒiv. A teaspoonful every hour.

We employ it with very marked advantage in the treatment of infantile pneumonia, associated with Aconite and Veratrum. In some cases, the prescription of Ipecac alone will be sufficient to arrest the disease in two or three days, especially if given in the first stages. It is also employed with excellent results in diseases of the respiratory apparatus of the adult.

We prescribe it in all cases of muco-enteritis. If there is little constitutional disturbance, Ipecac is used alone; if there is some hardness and increased frequency of the pulse, it is given in combination with Aconite.

We employ it in Dysentery, especially in the sporadic form from cold. The simple prescription of Ipecac is frequently successful, but with much febrile action it is associated with a sedative.

In small doses we employ it as a stimulant to the entire digestive tract, associating it with the bitter tonics, or the restoratives. For this purpose, it will prove very valuable, especially where there is some gastro-intestinal irritation.

IPOMÆA JALAPA.
(JALAP.)

So far as I know, this remedy has only been employed as a cathartic. It would be well to test it in doses so small that no cathartic action would follow; some desirable property might be developed.

14

IRIS VERSICOLOR.
(BLUE FLAG.)

We find the Iris described in our Dispensatory as "among the most valuable of our medicinal plants," "termed the *mercury* of Eclectic practice," and yet I am safe in saying that there has not been a good article in the market for a dozen years. The dried root of the drug trade possesses no more medicinal property than sawdust, and preparations from it, whether in the form of fluid extract or *Irisin*, are an imposition.

We would prepare a tincture from the fresh root, using Alcohol of 76°. There are two varieties of it, and that should be selected which presents a bluish mottled color on incision.

When prepared as above, the Iris is one of our best remedies. It is directly stimulant to waste and excretion, and also influences the lymphatic system. It may, therefore, be employed in all diseases in which there is bad blood, and imperfect nutrition. I regard it as one of our most certain remedies in the treatment of secondary syphilis.

It exerts a specific influence in cases of enlargement of the thyroid gland, and has effected cures in very severe cases. Here, as in other cases, we employ it uncombined, giving it internally, and using it as a local application. The dose of the tincture of Iris will vary from five drops to ℨj.

JEFFERSONIA DIPHYLLA.
(TWINLEAF.)

Preparation.—Prepare a tincture from the recent root, ℥viij. to Alcohol 76° Oj. Dose from gtt. j. to gtts. xx.

The Jeffersonia is a stimulant to mucous membranes, increasing their circulation, and checking profuse secretion. It may be employed in any case where these influences are desirable, and will give satisfaction. It exerts a feebly stimulant influence upon the skin, sufficient, however, to make it useful in chronic skin diseases. It is also claimed to be diuretic and anti-rheumatic. The remedy requires study, and may develop valuable properties.'

JUGLANS CINEREA.
(BUTTERNUT.)

Preparation.—Prepare a tincture from the fresh inner bark, in the proportion of ℥viij. to Alcohol 76° Oj. Dose from a fraction of a drop to five drops.

In minute doses, the Juglans exerts a marked influence upon the skin, and may be employed in either acute or chronic skin disease. Its influence in this direction requires study.

It also allays irritation of mucous membranes, and promotes their normal function. In some cases of intestinal dyspepsia, it will be found to give much better results than the bitter tonics.

A valuable laxative may be formed by making a watery extract of the Juglans, adding some aromatic to render it pleasant. I have a distinct recollection of the use of Butternut extract in the olden time to cure ague. It was given in large doses, and the catharsis would last for days, its influence being so constant and powerful that the patient would not have inclination or time to shake. In small doses, it leaves the bowels in a soluble condition, and is one of the few cathartics that may be employed to overcome obstinate constipation. *+ pecr . ratue ti peristalsis.*

JUNIPERUS SABINA.
(SAVIN.)

Preparation.—Prepare a tincture from the Savin, in the proportion of ℥viij. to Alcohol 76° Oj. Dose from gtt. j. to gtts. v.

Thus prepared, the Savin is a stimulant. It may be employed in menorrhagia, and in atonic leucorrhœa, with advantage. It may also be used as a stimulant in vesical catarrh, and in diseases of the urethra. In some cases of amenorrhœa it may be employed as a stimulant, but never in those cases presenting excitement of the circulation.

KALMIA LATIFOLIA.
(SHEEP LAUREL.)

Preparation.—Prepare a tincture from the recent leaves, in the proportion of ℥viij. to Alcohol 76° Oj. Dose from a fraction of a drop to five drops.

This is a favorite remedy of Prof. King, and he describes its use as follows: "It is an efficient remedy in primary or secondary syphilis, and will likewise be found invaluable in febrile and inflammatory diseases, and hypertrophy of the heart, allaying all febrile and inflammatory action, and lessening the action of the heart. In active hemorrhages, diarrhœa, and dysentery, it has been employed with excellent effect. I have extensively used this agent, and regard it as one of the most efficient agents in syphilis; and have, likewise, found it very valuable in inflammatory fevers, jaundice, and ophthalmia, neuralgia and inflammation."

I have employed it in secondary syphilis and atonic chronic inflammations with marked advantage, but have not used it for other purposes. Will some of our readers test it in the treatment of fever and inflammation to determine its analogy to the sedatives?

LAURUS SASSAFRAS.
(SASSAFRAS.)

A very good preparation of the Sassafras for office use, is a tincture of the bark of the root by percolation, using dilute alcohol or whisky. It forms a pleasant vehicle for many remedies, when we desire the gently stimulant and astringent action of the remedy. Tincture of Podophyllum added to it, in the proportion of ℨij. to ℥iv., in teaspoonful doses four times a day, forms an admirable alterative.

In the treatment of secondary syphilis, especially when manifesting itself in disease of the skin, the infusion will be found preferable. In this case I would direct an infusion of Sassafras with a small portion of Podophyllum, ℥ss. of the first, grs. x. of the second, to the pint of water, three times a day. It may be associated with the vapor bath, spirit-vapor bath, or sulphur bath in stubborn cases.

LARIX AMERICANA.

The American Larch deserves study, not in combination, as it has been employed, but singly, to determine its real medicinal value. For this purpose a tincture may be prepared from the recent bark, in the proportion of ℥viij. to Alcohol, 80° Oj. It has been employed in combination for a large number of diseases, but its influence upon mucous membranes and upon the skin, is probably most definite.

LAVANDULA VERA.
(LAVENDER.)

Lavender is the child's stimulant, and nothing, so far as I am aware, exercises so kindly an influence upon the digestive apparatus and the nervous system. A tincture may be formed of Oil of Lavender, ℥ij.; Dilute Alcohol, Oj. But the *Compound Spirit* will probably answer the needs of most physicians. I would like to test a tincture of the fresh herb, and if any of our readers are so located as to grow it,

and prepare such tincture, we will be obliged if they
will report.

LEONURUS CARDIACA.
(MOTHERWORT.)

Prepare a tincture from the fresh root, with dilute
Alcohol in the usual proportions. The line of experiment will be to determine its influence upon
the reproductive organs, and upon the nervous system. The dose may vary from five drops to ʒj.

LEPTANDRA VIRGINICA.
(BLACK ROOT.)

For general use prepare a tincture of the Leptandra, ℥viij. to Oj., using Alcohol of 50°. For some
purposes the infusion would be preferable, but is so
nauseous that most persons object to it. The dose
of the tincture as above will vary from gtts. ij. to
gtts. xx.

The Leptandra exerts a gentle stimulant influence
upon the entire intestinal tract, and its associate
viscera, and in medicinal doses strengthens functional activity. Its action in this direction is so persistent that it might be called a gastro-intestinal
tonic. There are some functions not well understood, as of the liver and spleen, and it would not
much improve our knowledge to say that it acted
upon these. But it exerts a marked influence in
those diseases in which there is enfeebled portal
circulation, and tendency to stasis of blood. Thus

in some cases of typhoid fever occurring in malarial localities the Leptandra has proven a very valuable medicine.

We do not believe there is any remedy that acts upon the *liver*, according to the old idea of medicine. It has been conclusively proven that preparations of Mercury do not, and that Podophyllin does not; and it is probable that we will have to give up the idea of cholagogues entirely. There is no doubt in my mind, however, that Leptandra does influence the function of the liver; not always to increase secretion of bile, but rather to bring the organ back to normal functional activity, whatever may have been the deviation.

Associated with the milder bitter tonics the Leptandra improves the digestive function, and stimulates normal excretory action from the bowels. This latter influence sometimes makes it a valuable adjunct to those remedies called alterative.

It has been employed in the treatment of intermittent fever with excellent results. Dr. Rolph writes, that "for many years my father's family employed it exclusively, and though living in a malarial region they were entirely exempt from ague. They used a tincture of the recent root, taking it before each meal." Quite a number of my acquaintances employ it after the chill has been broken with Quinine, and claim that its influence in preventing a recurrence is more decided than any other remedy.

LEPTANDRIN.

The best Leptandrin of the market is a *dried alcoholic extract*, the *strongest* is obtained by adding a portion of Podophyllum before tincturing. The resin is nearly worthless. The dried extract proves a very good remedy in many cases, and may be used for the same purposes as named for the tincture or infusion.

LIATRIS SPICATA.
(Button Snakeroot.)

Preparation.—Prepare a tincture from the recent root, ℥viij. to Alcohol 76° Oj. Dose from gtts. v. to ʒss.

The Liatris is gently tonic, and stimulates secretion from all the emunctories. Hence it has been added to various alterative combinations, and with some practitioners is very highly esteemed. It acts more directly upon the urinary apparatus, and probably upon the reproductive apparatus of both male and female.

LIQUIDAMBAR STYRACIFLUA.
(Sweet Gum.)

Some years since we had *sweet gum*, the exudation from this tree, recommended for the cure of asthma, and a number of cases from the South were given as proof. But experiments in the Northern States were not favorable. I judge, however, from some reports of Southern physicians, that the recent bark

15

contains valuable medicinal properties, as does the fresh exudation. For experiment I would suggest the preparation of a tincture from the fresh bark, using Alcohol of 76°. Its influence is probably most marked on mucous membranes, and probably it influences innervation from the pneumogastric and from the spinal cord.

LIRIODENDRON TULIPIFERA.
(YELLOW POPLAR.)

Preparation.—Prepare a tincture from the fresh root bark of the *Yellow Poplar*, using dilute Alcohol. Dose from gtts. v. to ℨj.

The great abundance and wide distribution of these trees, and the ease with which it may be obtained and prepared, and the really valuable character of the remedy, should bring it into general use. It is stimulant and tonic to the digestive apparatus, improving digestion and blood making. It also exerts an influence upon the nervous system, strengthening innervation and relieving those symptoms called nervous.

LOBELIA INFLATA.
(LOBELIA.)

Preparation.—Prepare a tincture from the ground seed, ℨviij. to Alcohol 98° Oj. Dose, from the fraction of a drop to ten drops.

The common use of Lobelia as an emetic is so well known that little need be said about it. In the form of the Compound Powder of Lobelia, or the Acetous Emetic Tincture of the Dispensatory, it gives us our most valued emetic when properly used. To obtain the curative effects of a lobelia emetic, the remedy should be given in small quantities frequently repeated, as it can be absorbed from the stomach, so that emesis when it does occur shall be from the general influence of the remedy in the blood, and not from its local irritant influence upon the stomach. Many physicians fail to obtain the benefit they have reason to expect because of its improper administration; it is not absorbed, but simply irritates the stomach.

Lobelia as prepared above is one of the most powerful vital stimulants in the Materia Medica. It strengthens the circulation, improves innervation, and by its influence upon the sympathetic nervous system gives increased activity of all the vegetative functions. These influences come from minute doses, one drop or less. I usually prescribe it in this proportion: ℞ Tincture of Lobelia, gtts. x. to xx.; Water, ℥iv. A teaspoonful every one or two hours.

In some cases where there is necessity for a speedy action, as in cases of angina pectoris or neuralgia of the heart, I give one or two full doses of twenty drops.

This preparation of Lobelia is specific in difficult labor from rigid os, vagina, or perineum. It also stimulates the contractile function of the uterus, and thus strengthens the pains. This use of Lobelia will be greatly prized when known. In tardy or difficult labor add ℨj. of the tincture to ℥iv. of water, and give a teaspoonful every fifteen minutes until slight nausea is produced, then in smaller quantities. In rigid os or perineum, I frequently employ it in the same way, and with excellent results, but in other cases give it in larger doses until nausea is induced.

Lobelia is a *sedative*, occupying a place between Veratrum and Aconite. I would be glad if each reader would put the tincture of the seed in his pocket case and employ it in fevers and inflammations in the same doses in which he uses Veratrum. I think it will prove very valuable, especially where there is necessity for stimulation.

LYCOPUS VIRGINICUS.
(BUGLE WEED.)

Preparation.—Prepare a tincture from the fresh plant gathered in July and August at the time of flowering, using ℥viij. to Alcohol 76° Oj.

The tincture of Lycopus prepared as above, will be found a very valuable remedy, and will take place with Veratrum and Aconite. It is a very certain sedative, where increased frequency of pulse is dependent upon want of power. For this purpose we employ it in all forms of chronic disease with frequent pulse, and in the advanced stages of acute disease where there is great debility. No remedy is more certain in its action in these cases; and we will find that as the pulse is reduced in frequency, it is increased in strength, and there is a more regular and uniform circulation of blood.

The remedy evidently acts upon the sympathetic system of nerves, and we not only have an improvement in the circulation, but every vegetative function feels its influence. Thus it improves the appetite and blood-making, nutrition and secretion.

It has been employed more extensively in the treatment of hemoptysis than in any other disease. In these cases its action is slow, but very certain, and its influence seems to come from its sedative action—in this it resembles Digitalis. Employed in phthisis, we find it relieving the cough, checking night sweats and diarrhœa, lessening the frequency of the pulse, improving the appetite and giving better digestion. We observe the same influence from the protracted use of Veratrum in these cases, evidencing the relationship between the remedies.

Those who live where the Bugle weed can be gathered, should not neglect the opportunity of procuring the fresh plant and preparing a tincture for the coming year. I am satisfied that it will well repay the trouble.

MAGNESIA, SULPHITE OF.

Sulphite of Magnesia was one of the anti-zymotic remedies recommended by Prof. Polli. We find in all that class of acute diseases which develop *typhoid*

... a need for remedies
... process in the blood.
... employed Sulphite of
... have found marked advan-
... in other cases, presenting
... similar ... symptoms it has done no
... in the harm.

... Sulphite ... Soda is indicated where
the tongue ... broad ... and covered with a pasty
... In these cases it will rarely disappoint
the practitioner.

But we have used the same ... the remedies
in cases in which the tongue is deep-red or dusky,
whether covered with a brown fur, or presenting
the ... glistening appearance noticed in some
of the more severe cases of typhoid fever, or typhoid
... Whenever the tongue is thus dark-red,
we can not give the Salt of Soda, for there is present
a ... indication for the use of an acid. We
may use Sulphurous Acid as the antiseptic, but frequently it is not well borne by the stomach.

In these cases the Sulphite of Magnesia will be
found an admirable remedy. We may say that it
may always be administered when the tongue is
dark-red, and shows a dark fur, and there is need
for a remedy to antagonize the septic process in the
blood. It is given in doses of grs. x. to grs. xxx.,
repeated every three hours.

MACROTYS RACEMOSA.
CIMICIFUGA RACEMOSA.
(BLACK COHOSH.)

Prepare a tincture from the fresh root gathered in September, using ℥viij. to Alcohol 76° Oj. Dose from the fraction of a drop to ten drops.

For years I have employed Macrotys as a specific in rheumatism, and with excellent success. Not that it cures every case, for it does not, neither would we expect this, for this would be prescribing a remedy for a name. Rheumatism may consist of varied pathological conditions, though in all there is the special lesion of the nervous system, which characterizes the disease. In one case we find the indications for the use of an Acid prominent, and this becomes a remedy for rheumatism. In another there are symptoms showing the need of Alkalies, and they prove curative.

Macrotys influences the nervous system directly, relieves rheumatic pain, when not the result of inflammation, and probably corrects the diseased condition (formation of lactic acid?) which gives origin to the local imflammatory process. Thus in the milder cases, where the disease has not localized itself as an inflammation, Macrotys is very speedy and certain in action. In rheumatic fever it is also positive in its action, and with the special sedatives gives excellent results. Where rheumatism has localized itself in an inflammatory process,

all the benefit we attain from it is, that we remove
the cause, and hence the reason for a long continuance of the inflammation.

It is a remedy for all pain having a rheumatic
character, and for this we prescribe it with the best
results. Those cases which go under the name of
rheumatic-neuralgia, are very speedily relieved by
it. In some cases the pains of weeks' duration disappear in a single day. Whilst the continuance of
the remedy will not unfrequently effect a cure in
these cases, in many it will require the additional
means necessary to give healthy functional activity
to some organ or part especially impaired.

The Macrotys influences directly the reproductive
organs. This influence seems to be wholly upon
the nervous system, relieving irritation, irregular
innervation, and strengthening *normal* functional
activity. For this purpose it is unsurpassed by any
agent of our Materia Medica, and is very largely
used.

Its influence is very marked in functional disease
of the reproductive organs of women. Associated
with Pulsatilla it is specific in many cases of dysmenorrhœa; it should be given for three or four
days before the expected period, and continued
until the flow is free. In amenorrhœa it is also one
of our most efficient agents. In rheumatism of the
uterus, to relieve false pains, or the many unpleasant
sensations attending pregnancy, it has no equal in
the Materia Medica.

Like all other *direct* remedies, it may be employed

in any case, no matter what name the disease may
have in our nosological classification, if the condition of the nervous system calls for it. The heavy,
tensive, aching. pains are sufficiently characteristic
and need not be mistaken. So prominent is this
indication for the remedy, in some cases (not rheumatic), that I give it with a certainty that the entire
series of morbid processes will disappear under its
use.

I had a very marked example of this in the severe
typho-malarial fever of this Fall. In one case, the
disease had continued through the first week, growing worse daily under the treatment adopted, until
the remarks of a night-watcher called my attention
to these pains. Questioning elicited the fact that
muscular pains had been severe from the first—but
the patient "thought it was part of the disease, and
there was no use to complain." The treatment
was changed from Veratrum and the Alkaline
Sulphites, to Aconite and Macrotys, and the patient
was convalescing in four days—there was marked
relief in twelve hours.

This will serve as an illustration of the fact,
"that a certain condition of disease may have that
prominence in a case, that an entire series of
morbid phenomena will pass away when it is removed;" or, in other words, that a single remedy
may prove curative, when a disease is complex—
removing the first in a series of morbid processes,
the others disappear of themselves.

MURIATE OF AMMONIA.

"Muriate of Ammonia is one of those common-
place and unattractive substances which we, in this
country, are little apt to credit with extensive remedial properties in disease."; We quote the first
sentence of an eminently suggestive paper by Dr.
Anstie (The Practioner, December, 1868), which
treats principally of the employment of this remedy for the relief of (1) various kinds of pain, and
(2) of certain cases of suspended secretion dependent on nervous exhaustion.   Before very briefly
describing some of the applications mentioned, we
think it right to state that we are by no means
prepared to coincide in Dr. Anstie's therapeutics,
in so far as this is founded on physiological data.
Under the first class the disease termed *myalgia* is
said to be specially amenable to treatment by
Muriate of Ammonia.   Doses of from ten to twenty
grains are recommended, and by their use this
disease may be cured as certainly as ague by quinia.
This class also includes various neuralgias proper,
such as migraine (usually referred to disorders of
digestion) and clavus hystericus; both of which
Dr. Anstie believes to be distinct and primary neuralgias of the fifth cranial nerve.   Of all the internal remedies that can be employed in these
headaches, none is apparently so beneficial as the
Muriate of Ammonia, its virtue depending on its
mildly stimulant properties.   It should be given in
the same doses as for myalgia.

MAGNOLIA.

The Magnolia Glauca and Accuminata possess tonic and stomachic properties, which may prove useful in medicine. Will some of our Southern readers prepare a tincture from the recent bark, and test it thoroughly. It may not prove better than a dozen similar articles, and yet supply a very good medicine to those who live where it is abundant.

MARRUBIUM VULGARE.
(HOARHOUND.)

Preparation.—Prepare a tincture from the fresh plant when in flower, using ℥viij. to Alcohol 76° Oj. Dose from gtts. j. to gtts. x.

The Hoarhound exerts a marked influence upon the respiratory apparatus. It is stimulant to all mucous surfaces, but especially to the laryngeal and bronchial, and it may be employed for this purpose. But it evidently has an action beyond this, and influences the function of respiration. Any one who has employed it will have seen this very marked in some cases. Let us have it thoroughly tried, and it may be another instance of a very valuable remedy, in a common article.

MARUTA COTULA.
(MAYWEED.)

In testing these indigenous remedies, will some one prepare a tincture from the fresh May weed and give it a thorough trial? The direction of the investigation will be shown by reference to the Dispensatory or Materia Medica.

MENISPERMUM CANADENSE.
(YELLOW PARILLA.)

The Yellow Parilla has been considerably employed for the indefinite purpose of an alterative. We have the testimony of the Dispensatory that: "In small doses, no obvious effects are produced on the general system." It may be worth while, however, to examine it further, and it will offer a good subject of study to some of our readers.

For experiment, prepare a tincture from the fresh root, ℥viij. to Alcohol 76° Oj. Use it in doses of from gtts. v. to ℨj.

MENTHA VIRIDIS.
(SPEARMINT.)

Preparation.—Prepare a tincture from the fresh herb, ℥viij. to Alcohol 76° Oj. Dose from gtts. v. to ℨj.

Mentha Viridis is not only a stimulant, but is one of the most kindly of the aromatics, and is rarely rejected by the stomach. As a stimulant, it will furnish a cheap and pleasant vehicle for many medicines.

But it is more than this. I regard it as one of the most certain of the vegetable diuretics, and employ it frequently for this purpose. In suppression of urine in children, a teaspoonful of the tincture is added to two ounces of water, sweetened, and given freely. So certain is its action in childhood, that I rarely think of giving anything else, except in cases where there is great irritation of the nervous system, and then Gelseminum is added to it in the usual doses.

MITCHELLA REPENS.
(PARTRIDGEBERRY.)

Preparation.—Prepare a tincture from the fresh plant, ℥viij. to Alcohol 76° Oj. Dose from gtts. v. to ℨss.

The Mitchella exerts a direct influence upon the reproductive apparatus of the female, giving tone and improving functional activity. It has been extensively used as a uterine tonic, to promote menstruation, to remove false pains and unpleasant sensations in the latter months of pregnancy, and has been thought to be a good preparative to labor, rendering the birth of the child easier, and less liable to accidents.

Many have failed to obtain these influences from the use of the common preparation "Compound Syrup of Partridgeberry," because it was prepared from old materials. If made from the green plant, as named above, we think it will give satisfaction.

ELATERIUM.

The common use of Elaterium, as a hydragogue cathartic is well known. I desire to call attention again to its direct action as described by Prof. King in the Eclectic Medical Journal, January, 1870, page 16. He claims that it is specific for " Chronic Inflammation of the Neck of the Bladder." Since the article was published I have received reports from two physicians as to its efficiency. He prepared the tincture by adding one drachm of Elaterium to one pint of Alcohol. Dose, half a fluid drachm three times a day until it acted upon the bowels, then six or eight drops.

MANATROPA UNIFLORA.
(Ice Plant.)

Will some of our subscribers prepare a tincture from the Ice-plant, and test it in the cases named in the Dispensatory. We especially want to know its influence upon the nervous system, and its action as a sedative. It is claimed to be remedial in convulsions, epilepsy, chorea, etc.

MYRICA CERIFERA.
(BAYBERRY.)

Preparation.—We prepare a tincture from the recent bark, in the proportion of ʒviij. to Alcohol 76° Oj.

As the Bayberry deteriorates unless carefully kept, it would be better to test a tincture of the fresh bark of the root. The dose will range from gtt. j. to ʒss.

I do not know that anything can be added to what is known of this agent. It has been extensively employed as a general stimulant, and as a special stimulant to mucous membranes, and with excellent results. Thomson recommended it in all cases where there was increased secretion from mucous membranes, whether it was catarrh or sore throat, bronchitis, disease of stomach or intestinal canal, or leucorrhœa.

It is in these cases especially that it will be found of advantage. I have employed it in chronic gastritis in small doses, associated with minute doses of Lobelia, with good success. The same combination will prove very valuable in typhoid fever, in typhoid dysentery, and in diarrhœa with increased mucous secretion.

The tincture prepared as above, will furnish a much better form for dispensing, as well as a more reliable remedy than much of the powder sold, and when once used, will become a prominent agent in the Office and the pocket case.

MOMORDICA BALSAMINA.
(Balsam Apple.)

The Balsam Apple is an annual climbing plant, grown in our gardens for its fruit, which is employed in domestic practice as a vulnerary, and an application to old sores, chapped hands, piles, etc. It is commonly prepared for use with alcohol or whisky. It evidently possesses medicinal properties, and I have seen good effects from its local use.

It is claimed to be poisonous when taken internally, yet I have known it taken with safety in doses of ten to thirty drops. Cures of dropsy are reported from its use. The limited use I have known made of it internally, was to relieve muscucular pains, lame back, and stiffness of joints; in some cases it seemed to do good. As the agent is very common, and easily cultivated, it would be well to prepare a tincture from the fresh fruit ℥viij. to Alcohol 76° Oj., and test it thoroughly, both as a local remedy, and used internally. Of such a preparation the dose would be quite small, say commencing with one drop.

NABALUS ALBUS.
(Lion's Foot).

Preparation.—Prepare a tincture from the fresh plant, ℥viij. to Alcohol 76° Oj. Dose from gtt. j. to gtts. xx.

This remedy has been but little employed. It was claimed to be specific to the poison of the rattlesnake, and to have been used with much success. It influences the nervous system directly, and experiment may develop a valuable use for it. It is not in the market, and we will therefore have to depend upon those who can procure it green, to determine its properties.

NEPETA CATARIA.
(CATNIP.)

Preparation.—Prepare a tincture from the fresh herb when in blossom, ℥viij. to Alcohol 76° Oj.

Catnip is a feeble remedy, and yet is as good as many in general use. Employed in the form named it will give satisfaction and well repay its preparation. It is a mild diaphoretic, but associated with the hot-foot bath, it will be found to place the skin in a soft moist condition, and relieve nervous irritation. It is especially to be recommended as a carminative for children. A teaspoonful added to four tablespoonfuls of hot water and sweetened, may be given freely, and is better than a tea of the dried herb.

NICOTIANA TABACUM.

Dr. Unziker, of this city, recommends the preparation of a tincture from the green plant, and its use as a sedative and in the treatment of diseases of the respiratory apparatus of children.

We value the local use of tobacco as a fomentation in cases of strangulated hernia, in some acute local inflammations, and in pseudo-membranous croup when the danger is imminent. It will also prove the best application to wounds and injuries where there are symptoms of tetanus.

In tetanus the alkaloid, Nicotine, has been employed with marked success, and it is probably our most certain remedy. It is given in doses of half to one drop, or if not tolerated by the stomach, it may be used by hypodermic injection. If the alkaloid can not be procured, an infusion may be used by mouth, by injection, or if not retained in sufficient quantity in these ways, it may be given by hypodermic injection.

Tobacco has been employed by the school of Rademacher, with reported success. It has also been employed to a limited extent in this country. The preparation advised is the "Aqua Nicotianæ Tabacum Spirituosæ Rademacheri," for which a formula is given.

This preparation is recommended highly in affections of the brain accompanying fever, in *rheumatismus acutus fixus et vagus*, in other affections of the brain and spinal marrow, in cholera morbus, and in cholera Asiatica.

To prepare it: Take of choice fresh green leaves of Nicotianæ Tabacum eight pounds, and cut them finely. Add of the best alcohol, by weight one and a half pounds, of distilled water as much as is necessary to distil over eight pounds (by weight) of the water.

The leaves are to be cut and the distillation effected immediately after they are pulled, with great care that there shall be no over-heating of the liquid, as, if the liquor be over heated it will have a very disagreeable odor of tobacco, which it does not have when the water is properly prepared.

Rademacher uses this water in every stage of the Asiatic cholera. In the earlier stages he gave the following: ℞ Aqua Puræ, f℥vij.; Soda Acet., ℨjss.; Aqua Nicotian., f℥j.; Gumi Arab., ℥ss. M.; dose, one tablespoonful every hour.

The great majority of cases treated with this mixture recovered immediately from the attack. In those cases where the attack was followed with a typhoid condition, he gave: ℞ Tinct. Ferri Acetici, f℥j.; Aqua Nicotian., f℥j.; Aqua Puræ, f℥vj.; Gumi Arabici, ℥j. M.; dose, one teaspoonful every hour.

NYMPHÆA ODORATA.

(White Pond Lily.)

Preparation.—Prepare a tincture from the fresh root of the White Pond Lily, in the proportion of ℥viij. to Alcohol 50° Oj. Dose from gtts. x. to ℥j.

My use of this remedy has been but limited, though from the reports of others, I deem it to possess decided medicinal properties. The general term *alterative* will express the kind of action that may be obtained from it. It exerts a special influence upon mucous tissues, and has been employed with advantage in diseases of the bronchiæ, the gastro-intestinal mucous surfaces, the bladder and the urethra. This will suggest the line of experiment, and we hope the remedy will be thoroughly tested and reported.

NITRIC ACID.

There are certain conditions in disease in which Nitric Acid is a very valuable remedy, and if it is possible to tell when it is indicated it will prove one of the most valuable of our specifics. I have been trying it for some months, and the following are the conclusions I have reached:

That there is a certain condition of stomach, in which there is irritability with enfeebled function, in which Nitric Acid is the remedy. That there is a lesion of digestion and blood-making other than the derangement of the stomach named, in which Nitric Acid is a direct remedy. That there is added to this, or separate from it in some cases, an impaired nutrition as well as a slow and imperfect retrograde metamorphosis of tissue and failure of excretion, in which Nitric Acid will prove a direct remedy.

Prof. E. Freeman informs me that he has employed it for some months in a class of stubborn ꞏ   ꞏting some of these features, with most marked success. His cases have embraced those of enfeebled digestion and blood making, and enfeebled and depraved nutrition. Taking some cases of scrofula, bad blood, and even phthisis.

There are four ways of determining the use of these remedies. The first employs them hap-hazard, in groups singly or combined, simply because they have been used in diseases covered by this name. The second is a better form of empiricism, and employs them one after another, in their supposed order of goodness, until some one hits the case in hand. The third generalizes the symptoms, and determines the quality of the lesion, and for this prescribes with some directness. The fourth tries to determine the principal lesion—basic lesion we have called it—by some positive signs or symptoms, and prescribes for this. Sometimes the prescription is in reality for a pronounced symptom, though if we would inquire far enough we might know there was a constant lesion underlying it.

In each of these four ways we may prescribe Nitric Acid; in the last two we may prescribe it in a rational manner.

I will not undertake to point out the evidences of the three pathological lesions, in which Nitric Acid has been employed with advantage, as our readers can read this up in our text-books; but I will hazard a guess as to the specific indication in certain instances:

If the tongue, whether pale, rose-red or deep-red, presents a violet haze, we have an indication for Nitric Acid. We will notice the same violet haze, wherever blood comes to the surface in the capillary circulation. I think we get the most decided results when the mucous membranes are moderately pallid. Don't mistake the deep, solid purple of the mucous membranes we see sometimes, for this violet-haze, for here the irritable stomach very frequently presents the red tip and edges of tongue, and sometimes elongated papillæ.

We do not use it for its acid properties, but probably the benefit is due to the supply of nitrogen in a peculiar form. Of course this is but a supposition.

I have treated successfully one case of inveterate chronic ague, two of malarial headache, and eight or ten of other diseases, and of course, in experimenting, mave missed it in quite as many cases. I have only the desire to call attention to the remedy, and have it thoroughly tested, asking that the symptoms be observed, so as to give us definite knowledge of the cases in which it will prove curative.

I prescribe it as follows : ℞ Nitric Acid, gtts. xxx.; Simple Syrup, ℥iv.; a teaspoonful every three hours.

NITRATE OF SODA.
(CUBIC NITRE.)

Pure Nitrate of Soda is a white salt, crystalizing in rhomboidal prisms; hence its common name—cubic nitre. It is soluble in three times its weight of cold water, giving a clear solution.

Given to the extent of two or three drachms in twenty-four hours it markedly increases the excretion of urea, and also influences secretion by skin and kidneys. Beyond this, it exerts a special influence upon the vegetative system of nerves, controlling irritation and inflammation.

It is held in high estimation by the school of Rademacher, as a remedy for dysentery, and also as a remedy in one of his three "epidemic constitutions of disease."

The indications for its use in acute diseases are: a swollen and puffed tongue, covered with a white or yellowish mucus; the mouth may be dry or moist, but the tongue must never show contraction, be elongated and pointed, or deep red. In other words, we must observe the general indications for the administration of an alkali.

Probably the special cases in which it will be found of most advantage are these: when the pulse is full, the surface flushed, slightly dusky or purplish; eyes injected, though not dry; an increased perspiration, though the skin remains hot.

The dose of Nitrate of Soda will range from ℨj. to ℥j. in the twenty-four hours; it is best given in solution, largely diluted with water.

POTASSÆ PERMANGANAS.

(PERMANGANATE OF POTASH.)

This salt, when pure, is in the form of slender prismatic crystals, of a dark purple color. It dissolves in five times its weight of water, the solution being a very dark purple. If this solution, in any preparation, shows a brownish or muddy tinge, the salt should be rejected. I am thus particular in describing its physical properties, for there has been a large amount of worthless material sold.

We use Permanganate of Potash principally as a local application where we have need of an antiseptic and stimulant. The indications for its use are, where the tissues are swollen from infiltration into the connective tissue. In cases of wounds, we will notice that the edges are swollen, and the process of repair stops. The infiltration continuing, the pus becomes watery and ichorous, granulations pale and flabby; the parts separate, and finally slough. In inflammation we have very nearly the same indications for its use—the inflammation always being of a low grade, and showing infitration of cellular tissue.

As a topical application, it will many times arrest the progress of carbuncle, felons, and like inflammations—a strong solution being employed. In a solution of ten grains to the ounce of water, it has ı used as an injection in gonorrhœa, to destroy irus; afterwards in the strength of two grains ʻ onnce, until the cure is complete.

OLEUM MORRHUÆ.
(COD LIVER OIL.)

We employ a bland and slightly odorous Cod-liver Oil in practice; probably Caswell & Mack's will give most satisfaction.

There is no doubt but benefit follows its use in appropriate cases, and sometimes the advantage is much greater than from the use of medicines. The principal indication for its use, is where an exalted temperature is maintained at the expense of the tissues. Cod-oil in such cases saves the tissues, and the burning of histogenetic food.

I employ it in cases of tuberculosis, scrofula, and in many forms of chronic disease, when the above indications exist. Especial attention is called to its use in local disease, with cacoplastic or aplastic deposits.

As the increased temperature is associated with increased frequency of pulse, we commonly associate it with Veratrum Viride. As a general rule the stomachic bitters are not advantageous at the same time. Many physicians fail to obtain advantage from the use of Cod-oil because they give tonics in excess at the same time.

ORIGANUM VULGARE.
(ORIGANUM.)

Preparation.—Prepare a tincture from the fresh herb, using ℥viij. to Alcohol 76° Oj. Dose, gtts. x. to ℨj.

This agent is a stimulant diaphoretic, and influences the reproductive organs of the female. It has been used in the treatment of colds, and in suppressed menstruation from cold.

OROBANCHE VIRGINIANA.
(BEECH DROPS.)

Beech drops contain a large proportion of tannic and gallic acids, and may be used for the general purposes of an astringent. I do not know that there is any advantage in taking a crude material that is scarce and high priced, when we can obtain its medical action from that which is common and cheap.

PÆONIA OFFICINALIS.

Preparation.—Prepare a tincture from the fresh root of the garden peony, in the proportion of ℥viij. to Alcohol 76° Oj. Dose from drops gtts. v. to ℨss.

This remedy has been but little used, yet the evidence is pretty conclusive that it possesses a marked influence upon the nervous system. It has been employed as an antispasmodic, and to relieve irritation of the nerve centers. Will some of our friends prepare a tincture in the summer and test it?

PANAX QUINQUEFOLIUM.
(GINSENG.)

Preparation.—Prepare a tincture from the fresh or recent root, in the proportion of ℥viij. to Alcohol 50° Oj. Dose from gtts. v. to gtts. xx.

We have laughed at the Chinese for their use of Ginseng, which we have deemed inert, but I am pretty well satisfied that in this, as in some other things, they have the advantage of us. A limited use of the article has given me a very favorable opinion of its influence.

Its first use, and a very important one, is in the treatment of nervous dyspepsia. I have obtained more benefit from it in my own person, than from any other remedy, and I have employed it with others with equal advantage. It exerts a decidedly beneficial influence in exhaustion of the brain from over work, and it is probable that its influence is as much in this direction as upon the stomach.

It is one of those remedies, however, that produces no marked improvement at first, and must be continued for weeks to obtain its good effects.

PAPAVER SOMNIFERUM.

Before describing the action of Opium, I want to draw the attention of my readers to the importance of having it good, and of not using Morphia as a substitute. Never buy Opium in powder, and in selecting the gum, take that which when broken gives the characteristic odor. Lastly, prepare your own tincture of Opium.

Opium in medicinal doses is a cerebral stimulant, and we will find this its most important use. From this stimulation comes sleep and rest to the nervous system.

In less degree it is a stimulant to the spinal-cord, and increases functional activity of all parts supplied from it.

Opium or its salts may be administered for the relief of pain, to produce sleep, or as a general stimulant to the vegetative processes, when the following conditions are present: A soft, open pulse, or where there is not the element of *hardness* and smallness; a soft (not dry) skin; a moist tongue; pallid face; and eyes dull, immobile or dilated pupils. It is contra-indicated, where there is a dry, contracted skin; small hard pulse; dry tongue; flushed face; bright eye, with contracted pupils.

There is no remedy that has been so much or so badly used as this. It is highly prized by the profession, and yet every physician can recall cases where its administration has proven injurious rather than beneficial. It has gained this extensive use because of the marked relief it gives from pain, and even though it fails so frequently, the successes are estimated, not the failures.

I believe the reader, by carefully studying the above indications and contra-indications, will be enabled to use the remedy so as to obtain its full palliative and curative action; not having the unpleasantness of failure to accomplish the desired object, or injury to the patient, to regret.

HYPODERMIC USE OF MORPHIA.—In this connection we may consider the advantages to be obtained from the hypodermic use of Morphia. It has been extensively employed for the relief of pain, and

many physicians would hardly practice medicine if
forced to give up their hypodermic syringes.

The advantages to be obtained from this use of
Morphia has not been over-estimated. But every
one who has employed it, will recollect cases of
failure, sometimes of injury, which were very mor-
tifying. Why the failure?

The indications for the hypodermic use of Morphia are the same as those just given for Opium,
and where there is present the contra-indications,
the use will not give the expected results, and may
prove injurious. Fortunately, in the majority of
cases of neuralgia, there is a soft, open pulse, the
cool pallid skin, and the evidence of an enfeebled
cerebro-spinal circulation. In such cases, the hypodermic use of Morphia gives present relief, and from
its topical stimulation, may effect a radical cure.

We never employ the hypodermic injection of
Morphia where there is a hard, small pulse, dryness
and constriction of skin, dry tongue, flushed face,
bright eyes and contracted pupils. He who uses it
in such cases, will very certainly be disappointed in
its action. In many cases of fever and inflammation, though the patient suffers pain, and the ordinary influence of Morphia in this way would be
very desirable, we withhold it.

PEROXIDE OF HYDROGEN.

Water receives an additional equivalent of oxygen, when it is presented to it in a nascent state. This combining with the hydrogen forms a deutoxide ($H O_2$.)

It was first brought to the notice of the profession by Dr. B. W. Richardson, of London, in 1860, and since has been used to a limited extent. He employed it in acute and chronic rheumatism, and in chronic inflammation with aplastic deposits. It improved digestion and nutrition, increased waste, oxidation and excretion.

PHOSPHORUS.

Preparation.—We prepare a tincture of Phosphorus, by taking ℥ij. to Alcohol 98° Oj.

The Phosphorus is divided under water, which being removed the Alcohol is poured on; it is allowed to stand for ten days, when it is ready for use. We use an excess of the Phosphorus, because in the commercial article there is but a small portion which can be acted upon by Alcohol. When of full strength, the tincture will contain about four grains to the ounce. We prepare it for use by adding one or two drachms of the tincture to four ounces of water, of which the dose will be one teaspoonful.

We employ this preparation of Phosphorus principally for its action upon the urinary and reproductive apparatus. It is especially useful to relieve vesical and prostatic irritation, especially when arising from or associated with sexual excess.

We also use it as a nerve stimulant. In some cases its influence will be quite marked, relieving irritation and improving nutrition.

THE HYPOPHOSPHITES.

The Hypophosphites, when well prepared, give us Phosphorus in the best form as a restorative. There is great difficulty, however, in obtaining reliable preparations, and many have been disappointed on this account.

I now use the *Compound Syrup of the Hypophosphites* (Gordon's), and it has given good satisfaction. It is especially useful when it is desirable to improve the nutrition of the nerve centers, though it exerts a favorable influence over the entire process of nutrition. I usually prescribe it in doses of a teaspoonful three times a day after meals. Its action is slow, like food, and time must be given to obtain its full benefit.

PHOSPHATE OF SODA.

We employ a pure article of Phosphate of Soda, and demand that it be finely powdered; probably Powers & Weightman's will give the most satisfaction.

The Phosphate of Soda has two uses—as a restorative, and for its influence upon the intestinal tract. As a restorative I employ it extensively with children, in those cases where there is impaired nutrition, with pallidity of tongue and mucous membranes. In these cases it will be found to exert a markedly beneficial influence. It is generally administered in milk in doses of one to three grains four times a day. We occasionally find a case in the adult where it will prove beneficial. These are uniformly marked by the pallid mucous membranes, and inaction of the bowels. The dose will vary from five to fifteen grains.

Its second use is as a laxative for children. We find cases of constipation that will yield to no remedies, the child suffers from indigestion, and occasionally from colic. In these cases Phosphate of Soda in doses of from three to five grains, three times a day, will give permanent relief.

Phosphate of Soda is also an excellent laxative for the adult, especially in cases of habitual constipation, with hardened feces. In this case twenty to thirty grains in a large glass of water, is taken on going to bed at night

PHYTOLACCA DECANDRA.
(POKE.)

Preparation.—We prepare a tincture from the fresh root, ℥viij. to Alcohol 76° Oj. Dose gtts. ij. to ℨss.

This is one of those remedies that loses its medical properties by drying, and the crude article furished from drug stores is wholly worthless, as are the preparations from it.

The tincture of the *fresh* root is one of my favorite remedies. It exerts a direct influence upon the processes of waste and nutrition, and therefore possesses those properties called alterative in a high degree. I have used it in secondary syphilis, in chronic skin disease, and in scrofula, with excellent results.

It has a direct influence upon the mammary glands, and will generally arrest inflammation if given in the early stage. I also employ it in cases of sore nipples, both internally and locally, with good results.

It has been considerably employed in diphtheria, and many believe it will be found a specific to the sore throat. In this disease it is given internally, and employed as a local application.

It will be found a very valuable remedy, and as it is so common, I would advise every one to prepare them a tincture in the fall and test it in practice.

PIPER NIGRUM.
(BLACK PEPPER.)

We make a tincture of Black Pepper in the proportion of ℥viij. to Alcohol 76° Oj. The Pepper should be finely ground and packed in the percolator, moistened with Alcohol and allowed to stand twenty-four hours, then run the remainder of the Alcohol through it. Dose, gtts. ij. to ℥j.

Black Pepper is a remedy I value very highly. As a gastric stimulant it certainly has no superior, and for this purpose we use it in congestive chills, in cholera morbus, and other cases of a similar character. In atonic dyspepsia it may be associated with Hydrastis or other stomachic bitter, or sometimes with Nux Vomica or Strychnia. I have used it associated with Tincture of Macrotys in atonic amenorrhœa with advantage, and sometimes the same combination will be found beneficial in dysmenorrhœa.

It may be used with excellent results in the treatment of intermittents, preparing the way for Quinia and associated with it. In these cases it is used in full doses.

PIX LIQUIDA.
(TAR.)

We prepare a glycerole of tar for local use in the following way: Heat a pound of glycerine and of tar in separate vessels; whilst heating, rub up an ounce of starch in a mortar with a portion of the glycerine, and stir it in until thoroughly mixed; when hot pour the two together, boil for a moment, then stir until cool.

Glycerole of tar prepared in this way is a specific for many forms of pruritus. In pruritus-ani it is so certain in its action, that I prescribe it with an almost positive certainty that it will not only give present relief, but will effect a radical cure. In eczema with pruritus, it has proven an admirable remedy, and has effected cures in protracted and very stubborn cases. The indication for its use is *itching*.

Tar has been used internally, with reported good effects. To test it in chronic bronchial disease, and for the relief of cough, I would suggest one part of tar to nine parts of glycerine, combined with heat.

PLANTAGO CORDATA.
(WATER PLANTAIN.)

Preparation.—Prepare a tincture from the fresh root, ℥viij. to Alcohol 76° Oj. Dose from gtts. x. to ℨss.

This remedy has been but little used, yet from what we know of it, we think it deserves careful investigation. It exerts a direct influence upon the nervous system, allaying irritation and giving better innervation. It was employed in the cholera of 1832 with marked success, and Prof. Jones thinks it likely to prove one of the most certain remedies we have in that disease. Let some of our physicians prepare the remedy, and report.

PODOPHYLLUM.
(MAY APPLE.)

For common use, prepare a tincture from the root in the proportion of ℥viij. to Alcohol 76° Oj. Dose gtt. j. to ℨss.

I am satisfied that a trial of a tincture of Podophyllum will satisfy any one that it is preferable to Podophyllin in general practice. It makes no difference whether it is to be used as a stimulant to the digestive tract, as an alterative, for its general cathartic effect, or as an emeto-cathartic.

For its stimulant influence and to improve digestion, I frequently use it in combination with the stomachic bitters, or Nux Vomica, Quinia, and Iron; necessarily the dose is small. As an alterative, *a remedy to increase waste*, it may be combined with other agents that act in the same direction, with the bitter tonics and restoratives, or many times with Veratrum. A common prescription of mine is: ℞ Tincture of Veratrum, ʒss.; Tincture of Podophyllum, Tincture of Nux Vomica, aa ʒj.; Water, ʒiv. A teaspoonful every four hours. In place of water, the vehicle may be simple syrup or glycerine, a tincture of Mentha Viridis or of Amygdalus. The case in hand will suggest the best vehicle.

I am well satisfied that in small doses, associated with the bitter tonics and restoratives and good food, it is decidedly the best remedy we have in the treatment of old syphilitic lesions. Its action may be greatly aided sometimes by the use of the vapor-bath, or by sulphur and iodine baths.

For common use in malarial fevers, where the tongue is uniformly coated yellow, I would suggest its combination with Veratrum and Aconite, as in the following: ℞ Tincture of Veratrum, gtts. xx.;

Tincture of Aconite, gtts. x.; Tincture of Podophyllum, ʒss. to ʒj.; Water, ℥iv. A teaspoonful every hour.

For the ordinary routine of medicine, as a cathartic, combine it with neutralizing cordial, as ℞ Tincture of Podophyllum, ʒij. to ℥ss.; Compound Syrup of Rhubarb, ℥jss. A teaspoonful every two or three hours. The addition of a small portion of Tinctures of Lobelia or Ipecac will render its action more efficient and kindly. As an emeto-cathartic give it with a ginger-tea, or other stimulant taken freely.

PODOPHYLLIN.

To obtain the direct action of Podophyllin, we prepare it for use by thorough trituration with sugar of milk or white sugar. I prefer the trituration one part of Podophyllin to one hundred of sugar.

The specific use of Podophyllin in this form is to arrest increased mucous secretion from the small intestine and give it power to perform its function. It will cure acute or chronic diarrhœa with mucous discharges, and in some cases of cholera infantum it "acts like a charm." No one who has used the trituration of Podophyllin in these cases would be willing to dispense with it, and many will find it of advantage in other cases.

POLEMONIUM REPTANS
(JACOB'S LADDER.)

This remedy has been but little used, yet it might repay study. If some of our friends will prepare a tincture from the fresh root and test it, we would be glad to hear the report.

POLYGALA SENEGA.
(SENEGA.)

Preparation.—Prepare a tincture from the recent dried root, ℥viij. to Alcohol 50° Oj. Dose, gtts. ij. to gtta. xx.

The stimulant influence of Senega upon the throat and bronchial mucous membrane is well known, and is probably its most important use. For this purpose I prefer to use it in the form of tincture to that of syrup so commonly employed. In chronic bronchitis with profuse secretion, it may be combined with small doses of Ipecac and Veratrum.

Its influence upon the kidneys and reproductive organs needs to be studied, and I have no doubt some important uses will be found for it. I have employed it in squamous disease of the skin, and like its action very much; it is one of a very few remedies that influence these diseases.

POLYGONUM PUNCTATUM.
(Water Pepper.)

Preparation.—Prepare a tincture from the fresh herb, in the proportion of ℥viij. to Alcohol 76° Oj. Dose gtts. ij. to ℥ss.

I regard the tincture of Water-Pepper as one of our most certain stimulant diaphoretics. It is also one of the best emmenagogues, especially when the arrest is from cold. It influences the urinary and reproductive organs, but its action in these directions needs to be studied.

POLYPODIUM VULGARE.
(Polypody.)

This remedy is now but little used, yet will probably repay study. For experiment, a tincture should be prepared from the fresh root with dilute alcohol, in the usual proportion.

POLYTRICHUM JUNIPERUM.
(Hair-Cap Moss.)

The hair-cap moss has been especially employed as a diuretic, and so long as it could be readily procured without admixture, gave good satisfaction. I do not know that it has any direct influence, other than to increase the secretion of water in the urine—a hydragogue diuretic; but it might be well to study its action more closely.

POPULUS TREMULOIDES.
(POPLAR.)

Preparation.—Prepare a tincture from the fresh bark of the white poplar, in the proportion of ℥viij. to Alcohol 76° Oj.   Dose ℨss. to ℥j.

This remedy is so common and may be so easily prepared, that it should come into more general use as a tonic and stomachic.   It improves the appetite and strengthens digestion, exerting its influence more especially upon the upper intestine.   It influences the urinary organs, but its action in this direction needs to be studied.

PRINOS VERTICILLATUS.
(BLACK ALDER.)

Preparation.—Prepare a tincture from the recent bark of the Black Alder, in the proportion of ℥viij. to Alcohol 50° Oj.   Dose from gtts. v. to ℨss.

This remedy is a stimulant to the digestive and blood-making organs, and may be advantageously employed for the general purposes of a tonic.   But beyond this, it influences the vegetative processes, probably through the sympathetic system of nerves, strengthening the circulation, aiding nutrition, and the removal of waste.   We have used it but little, yet the testimony in its favor is such, that we strongly recommend its trial.

PRUNUS VIRGINIANA.
(WILD CHERRY.)

The tincture of Prunus should be prepared from the fresh inner bark, in the proportion of ʒviij. to Alcohol 50° Oj. Dose from gtts. v. to ʒss.

In addition to its tonic influence, which it possesses in common with many of our indigenous bitters, it has other valuable medicinal properties. It allays irritation of mucous membrane, both of the gastro-intestinal canal, the respiratory tract, and urinary apparatus. This will probably prove its most important use. The influence upon the circulation and upon secretion is not decided, but in atonic states will sometimes be found very desirable. In some of these cases I have combined it with the Tincture of Nux Vomica or Solution of Strychnia, with excellent results.

The remedy is so common, and so easily prepared, that it should find a place in every office, and I have no doubt that as it is employed, other uses than those named will be developed.

PTELEA TRIFOLIATA.
(WAFER ASH).

Preparation.—Prepare a tincture from the bark of the root, ʒviij. to Alcohol 76° Oj. Dose gtts. x. to ʒss.

Ptelea is an excellent tonic, hardly surpassed in its general uses by any agent of our Materia Medica, if we except Hydrastis. It may be employed in all atonic states of the stomach and upper intestinal canal, when it is desirable to increase the appetite and digestion. It exerts a specific influence in some cases of asthma, giving present relief, and effecting permanent cures. I have used it in a considerable number of these cases, but can not give any symptoms which would lead me to prescribe this in preference to other remedies.

PTERIS ATROPURPUREA.
(ROCK BRAKE.)

A tincture should be prepared from the entire plant *fresh*, ℥viij. to Alcohol 76° Oj. Dose from gtts. v. to gtts. x.

This remedy has been but little used except in domestic practice. It exerts a marked influence upon the excretory apparatus, controlling diarrhœa, dysentery, night sweats, hemorrhages, etc. This may depend to some extent upon its tannic acid, but there is an influence beyond this. Will some of our practitioners prepare a tincture and test it, and report?

PETROLEUM.

There are two varieties—the *heavy* and the *light* coal-oils, which differ as much in their medicinal properties as they do in use—probably the heavy should alone be used.

A very pure and heavy oil, known as Mecca Oil from the well that yields it, is recommended. It is *a dark*, bland oil—not unpleasant to the taste, and *is* furnished by the gallon from our druggists at '2.00.

It has been employed with advantage in chronic bronchitis and laryngitis, and phthisis, with bronchial irritation. Some contend that for bronchial disease it is unsurpassed. It has also been employed in scrofula, chronic disease of the urinary apparatus, and in chronic skin diseases. It would be well to test it thoroughly in these cases, and also for its influence upon the nervous system. The dose will vary from one drop to a teaspoonful.

PROPYLAMIN.

The Propylamin of commerce is obtained from *herring pickle*, and is in the form of a colorless transparent liquid; the muriate is in the form of powder and is about two-thirds of its strength. We prepare it for use by adding twenty-four drops, or thirty-six grains of the Muriate of Propylamin to six ounces of mint water, the dose of which will be from a tea to a tablespoonful.

Investigation has determined that Propylamin is the same as the *Secalin* derived from Ergot. My use of the remedy clearly proved the analogy between the Propylamin and Ergot in its poisonous effects.

The remedy was introduced by Dr. Owenarius of St. Petersburgh, Russia, as a specific for rheumatism, and a large number of cases were reported in which it had proven curative in a short time. This was in 1856, and it was tested in this country as well as in Europe, but without very satisfactory results.

I employed it in quite a number of cases of rheumatism, and at first thought very favorably of its
action, but developing marked typhoid disease in
some cases I became alarmed and dropped it. I
am confident it possesses a marked influence upon
the animal economy, but unless used with care, it
is as likely to be for evil as good. I developed a
typical typhoid fever with it, that ran a course of
five weeks, with intestinal irritation, rose-colored
spots and typhomania. It was evidently due to the
medicine, as when its administration was commenced it was a case of simple inflammatory rheumatism about the fifth day, and there was no such
thing as typhoid fever that year.

In employing the Propylamin in the treatment
of rheumatism, I think it necessary to first bring
the circulation fully under the influence of the sedatives, and then establish secretion—now the remedy
may be used with safety.

In doses much smaller than named, I feel confident the Propylamin will be found a stimulant to
the entire vegetative functions. It strengthens the
circulation, improves nutrition, and stimulates
waste and secretion. In these directions it deserves
thorough investigation. The proportions I would
recommend would be gtts. v. to gtts. x. to mint
water ℥iv., a teaspoonful every three or four hours.
Or better, ℞ Muriate of Propylamin, grs. x.; Sugar
of Milk, grs. 1000; triturate thoroughly; dose one
to five grains.

PTEROSPORA ANDROMEDA.
(CRAWLEY.)

Preparation.—Prepare a tincture from the fresh plant and root, ℥viij. to Alcohol 76° Oj. Dose from gtts. j. to v.

The Crawley is a very scarce article, and in the market commands a high price. When the practitioner can obtain it and prepare it himself, he will find it one of the most valuable of the Materia Medica. It possesses decided sedative properties, and may be employed for this purpose, but its principal use is to establish waste and secretion. Following or associated with Veratrum or Aconite, there is no remedy that will more quickly and certainly establish secretion from skin and kidneys. It is probable that other uses will be developed by experiment.

PULMONARIA OFFICINALIS.
(LUNGWORT.)

Preparation.—Prepare a tincture from the fresh leaves, ℥viij. to Alcohol 50° Oj. Dose, from ten drops to ℥ss.

The Lungwort has a popular reputation as a remedy in diseases of the chest. It would be well to test it thoroughly and determine its medicinal action in this direction.

PULSATILLA NIGRICANS.
(PULSATILLA.)

We employ the German tincture prepared from the fresh herb according to the Homœopathic pharmacy. That prepared from the imported dried herb will not give good satisfaction. We usually prescribe it in this proportion: ℞ Tincture of Pulsatilla, ʒj. to ʒij.; Water, ℥iv. A teaspoonful every four hours.

The principal use of Pulsatilla is to relieve certain cerebral symptoms with difficulty relieved by other remedies. In some diseases of women, in spermatorrhœa and prostatorrhœa, in heart disease, and some other chronic affections, we find certain *head* symptoms playing an important part, and giving a good deal of trouble. The patient is nervous, restless, has an active imagination for disease, a fear of impending danger, etc. These symptoms are very unpleasant, and not unfrequently prevent the curative action of remedies. Pulsatilla reaches them and gives prompt and certain relief.

I would not treat some cases of spermatorrhœa without I could employ this remedy. For with the unnatural excitement of the mind, no remedy would exert a curative influence. So in some cases of heart disease, the head symptoms are the most prominent and unpleasant features. Relieve the unpleasant mental sensations and dread of danger, and we have removed a permanent cause of excitement.

Though Pulsatilla is the remedy for nervousness, it must not be given with any expectation of benefit when the excitement depends upon irritation and determination of blood. In this case it will either exert no influence or it will be unfavorable.

The Pulsatilla exerts a marked influence upon the reproductive organs of both male and female. I regard it as decidedly the best emmenagogue, when the suppression is not the result of or attended by irritation and determination of blood; where there is simple suppression from atony or nervous shock, it may be used with confidence. In male or female it lessens sexual excitement. It does not diminish sexual power, but rather strengthens it by lessening morbid excitement.

There are other uses for the remedy, but those I have named are prominent ones, and readily recognized. I value the remedy very highly, and am satisfied from an experience of ten years in its use that I do not overestimate it.

PYRETHRUM PARTHENIUM.
(FEVERFEW.)

Preparation.—Prepare a tincture from the fresh plant, ℥viij. to Alcohol 50° Oj. Dose from gtts. v. to ℨss.

The Feverfew has the reputation of being an admirable tonic, at the same time being one of the most pleasant of its class. It influences the entire intestinal tract, improves the appetite and digestion, and stimulates secretion. It also exerts an influence

upon the skin and kidneys.   This is one of the little
used medicines that deserves careful study, and as
it is cultivated in our gardens it is within the reach
of all.

PYROLA ROTUNDIFOLIA.
(False Wintergreen.)

Preparation.—Prepare a tincture from the fresh
plant, ℥viij. to Alcohol 50° Oj.   Dose from gtts. v.
to ʒss.

This also is likely to prove a valuable remedy and
deserves to be studied.   It has marked tonic properties, and exerts an influence upon the urinary
organs, relieving irritation.   It is claimed to exert
an influence upon the nervous system, and to have
been successfully employed in convulsions and
epilepsy.

PYRUS MALUS.
(Apple Tree.)

Preparation.—Prepare a tincture from the fresh
root-bark of the apple-tree, ℥viij. to Alcohol 76° Oj.
Dose from gtts. v. to ʒss.

Though so common and easily prepared, this
remedy has been but little studied.   It possesses
tonic and antiperiodic properties, and may be employed in a great many cases instead of more costly
remedies.   The only use I have made of it was in
intermittent fevers, and whilst it was not a substitute for Quinia, it evidently exerted a good influ-

ence upon the disease, especially in preventing a recurrence of the paroxysms.

QUERCUS RUBRA.
(RED OAK.)

The Red Oak is not only astringent from its tannic acid, but it possesses other properties that will render it useful in some cases. Among them is its tonic influence, and its action upon skin and kidneys. I have used it in chronic eczema associated with Rumex, both as a local and internal remedy, with marked advantage. A combination of Quercus Rubra, Rumex and Alnus is my favorite remedy in obstinate cases of scrofula where there are old ulcers, feeble tissues and cicatrices. In these cases I use it as a local application and as an internal remedy.

I have employed it principally in infusion and decoction, but for experiment would recommend the preparation of a tincture, ℥viij. of the fresh inner bark to Alcohol 76° Oj. Dose from gtts. v. to ℨss.

QUINIA SULPHAS.
(QUININE.)

There is no occasion to give a lengthy description of the *specific* action of Quinine, as every one of my readers is thoroughly conversant with it. But it may be of use to some, to state the conditions necessary to its kindly and medicinal action.

19

Probably there is no remedy in the Materia Medica that gives so many failures as this, and I think we may be safe in assuming that it is given ten times where its specific action is obtained once. Every one will recollect cases in which it did *not* break up periodic disease, many more cases in which its influence was but temporary, a large number in which it produced unpleasant cerebral symptoms, and some in which a Quinia disease was developed, which was much worse than the original malady.

Why is this? Is it the fault of the remedy, the fault of the patient, or the fault of the practitioner? O, the doctor answers, it is from *idiosyncrasy!* So we believe, but we locate the idiosyncrasy in the doctor's head, and not in the patient.

I have taught for years, that if we are to expect the kindly and curative action of Quinia, the stomach must be in condition to receive and absorb it, and the system in condition for its action. If we have a proper condition in these respects, we will hear nothing of roaring in the ears, vertigo, etc., but its action will be most kindly. The rule is very simple—*Given, a soft and open pulse, a moist skin, moist and cleaning tongue*, and Quinia will act kindly, antidote the malarial poison, or in small doses improve innervation. Always get this condition before prescribing the remedy, and you will never be disappointed in its action.

As an antiperiodic I believe in prescribing *single* doses. Put the stomach in proper condition, regulate the circulation, establish secretion, and then give *one* full dose of the remedy, (10 to 15 grs.) The best form of the remedy is in solution with one or two ounces of water, using a sufficient quantity of sulphuric acid.

This is not only the most certain method of administration, but I think it will be found the most pleasant.

It is hardly necessary to impress upon the reader the necessity of determining the periodic element in disease. Whilst we may not know what it is, or how Quinine antidotes it, we know that its removal cures, or at least paves the way to a cure.

But Quinine is not *specific* to all agues. We see it given day after day, week after week, in many cases, without any advantage. But on the contrary, it excites the nervous and vascular systems, and at last produces a chronic erythism of them, that is correctly named "the Quinine disease." From this, recovery is far more difficult than from the malarial affection.

Is it possible then, to determine the cases in which Quinine will prove specific, and the cases in which it will fail? I think it is. It antidotes the malarial poison only when kindly received and absorbed, and when the system is in such condition that it can be readily excreted. Given, the condition of pulse, skin and tongue, that we have already named, and its action is as certain as could be desired.

In some cases, the general treatment directed to obtaining normal activity of the various functions, is the most successful. In some cases Nux Vomica or Strychnia is preferable. In others minute doses of Arsenic antagonizes the malarial poison. Whilst in some rare cases, I have treated the disease most successfully with Aconite and Belladonna.

As a stimulant to the cerebro-spinal centers, its use is very important. In many forms of disease, especially in the advanced stages, we find an impaired innervation, preventing functional activity, or its restoration and continuance by the use of remedies. It is essential to success that innervation be increased, not temporarily by the use of stimulants, but somewhat permanently. This we accomplish by the administration of small doses of Quinine (grs. ½ to grs. ij). Even here, we find it necessary to observe the rules for its administration already noticed—the patient must be prepared for its use.

It favorably influences the nutrition of the nerve centres, and hence is employed in the treatment of chronic disease with enfeebled innervation, with marked advantage. There are two classes of chronic disease in which it is useful—the one in which there is a malarial influence, with obscure periodicity, and the other the enfeebled innervation, as named above.

Its general tonic and stomachic influence, (when obtained) is most certainly from this action upon the nervous system—the influence extending to the sympathetic ganglia, as well as to the cerebro-spinal centers. In some cases this action is very important, improving digestion and blood-making, and nutrition, as well as waste and excretion—aiding " the renewal of life."

POTASSII FERROCYANURETUM.
(PRUSSIATE OF POTASH.)

The Prussiate of Potash was omitted in its proper place by mistake. It is a remedy I value highly, and though little used it is certain to become a favorite.

We find it in market in the form of prismatic crystals of a clear lemon-yellow color, inodorous, possessed of a sweetish-bitter saline taste. If the salt is dirty, dark-colored, or parti-colored, it should be rejected. We prepare it for use by adding ℨss. to Water, ℥iv. Dose, one teaspoonful every three hours.

In chronic disease where there is marked irritability of the nervous system, with frequency of pulse, we will find it an excellent remedy. It lessens irritation of the nervous system, and acts as a special sedative to the circulation. In chronic disease of the reproductive organs in women, with hysterical manifestations, it exerts a direct and marked influence—so in hypochondriacal affections in the male.

It exerts a decided influence upon mucous membranes. When they are pallid, lax, and give increased secretion, the Prussiate of Potash may be used with advantage. It makes little difference, whether of nose, throat, bronchial tubes, intestinal mucous membrane, or chronic vaginitis with leucorrhœa, the influence is the same.

This will suggest to the practitioner the cases in which it may be tested: where there is excitation, but impaired nutrition of the nerve centres, and where there is feebleness of mucous membranes with increased secretion of mucus.

RANUNCULUS BULBOSUS.
(Crowfoot.)

Preparation.—Prepare a tincture from the fresh root in the proportion of ℥viij. to Alcohol 76° Oj. Dose, the fraction of a drop, very largely diluted with water. The remedy is exceedingly acrid, and must be used with care.

Prof. King reports the cure of nursing sore mouth by its internal administration in small doses in infusion. It has also been employed as a stimulant to the vegetative processes, with reported good results. It should be thoroughly tested, and we will be obliged to any one of our readers for a report. Prescribe it in about the following proportion: ℞ Tincture of Ranunculus, gtts. x.; Water, ℥iv. Dose, a teaspoonful.

RHAMNUS CATHARTICUS.
(Buckthorn.)

Two preparations of this agent may be used. Prepare a tincture from the fresh bark in the proportion of ℥viij. to Alcohol 50° Oj. Dose, gtts. vj to gtts. xxx. Prepare a tincture from the berries, in the proportion of ℥viij. to Alcohol 76° Oj. Dose, from the fraction of a drop to two to five drops, largely diluted with water.

Buckthorn berries have been employed as a cathartic, but their activity, attended with nausea, dryness of the throat, thirst and tormina, made their use limited. The tincture of the berries in small doses may be tested for its influence on the digestive apparatus, in diseases of the nose, throat, and respiratory organs, and as a stimulant to the vegetative processes.

It is claimed that a preparation from the bark gives one of the most efficient alteratives of the Materia Medica. Dr. William Goltry claimed that a tea made of the bark or berries would cure cancer and scrofulous diseases generally. Dr. William S. Knight writes, " I have been using the Rhamnus Catharticus in all forms of scrofulous disease for the last two years (1866) with good effect. I make an infusion from the bark and let the patient drink as much as he well can during the day, so as not to act too much upon the bowels."

RHEUM PALMATUM.
(RHUBARB.)

Preparation. — Prepare a tincture from the best Russian, Turkey, or India Rhubarb, in the proportion of ℥viij. to Alcohol 50° Oj. Dose, from the fraction of a drop to ten drops.

It is not worth while to speak of the common use

of Rhubarb, as there is no remedy better known
and more used. But it will be noticed that we
have recommended a wholly different preparation,
and we propose to dispense it in small doses for its
direct action.

In the proportion of ℞ Tincture of Rhubarb, ℥j.,
Water, ℥iv., a teaspoonful every half hour or hour,
it will be found one of our best remedies to control
irritation of the stomach, and arrest vomiting. In
children it is especially useful, where there is nervous irritability, manifested by restlessness, screams,
and convulsive contraction of muscles.

In the same doses, less frequently repeated, it
will prove an excellent tonic, strengthening the
functions of both stomach and intestines, giving
improved digestion. In indigestion, with some
diarrhœa, of a papescent character, it will be found
a good remedy.

In some cases it will prove our best remedy in the
treatment of obstinate constipation. The cases are
those in which there is an unnatural sensation of
constriction in stomach and bowels, and contraction
of the abdominal muscles. I prescribe it in these
cases in doses of ten drops in a large glass of water,
on rising in the morning. In the severer cases it is
associated with thorough fatty innunction over the
abdomen, and friction.

I employ it as a restorative, where there is special
need of increased nutrition of nerve tissue. It is
thus associated with the preparations of Phosphorus, and with Cod Liver Oil.

RHODODENDRON CHRYSANTHUM.
(RHODODENDRON.)

A tincture is prepared from the fresh leaves collected in September; that we employ is imported from Germany. Two native species—the R. Maximum and R. Punctatum possess similar properties, but much milder, and should be tested.

The influence of the Rhododendron on the circulation is very marked. It undoubtedly acts like Veratrum and Aconite, stimulating the circulatory apparatus through the sympathetic, and diminishing the frequency of the pulse by increasing the power of the heart, and removing capillary obstruction. Acting in this way, it has been employed with advantage in rheumatism, gout, syphilis, and some acute diseases. It is claimed to exert an influence upon the reproductive apparatus, being used in orchitis, in suppression of gonorrhœa, and in hydrocele. It has been but little employed in this country, but our native specimens deserve a thorough examination.

RHUS GLABRUM.
(SUMACH.)

Preparation.—Prepare a tincture from the fresh root bark, ℥viij. to Alcohol 76° Oj. Dose from gtts. v. to gtts. xx.

The Sumach as thus prepared exerts a direct influence upon the processes of waste and repair—alterative. It has not been much used, and we can

not tell whether it will prove better than others of
this class; still it deserves a thorough trial. It is
claimed to be antidotal to the action of mercury,
especially in chronic mercurial disease, and has
been employed in the treatment of secondary
syphilis, after mercurialization, with advantage.

RHUS TOXICODENDRON.
(Poison Oak.)

Prepare a tincture from the recent leaves, ℥viij.
to Alcohol 76° Oj. Added to water in the proportion of gtts. v. to gtts. x. to ℥iv., the dose is a
teaspoonful. The R. Radicans, R. Venenata, and
R. Pumilum may be prepared in the same manner,
and deserve a thorough investigation.

The Rhus is likely to prove one of our most
valuable medicines, and will be highly prized when
its use is learned. It is antidotal to such animal
poisons (zymotic) as determine to the skin, in erysipelas or erysipeloid disease, or in low grades of
inflammation of cellular tissue, or in low grades of
inflammation of mucous membranes. A frequent,
small pulse, redness of mucous membranes, brown
sordes, bright superficial redness of skin, tympani-
tis, acrid discharges from bowels or bladder, are indications for its use. So also is inflammatory action,
presenting tumid, bright reddened tissues, deep
seated or superficial burning pain, inflammation
giving an ichorous discharge, in which the tissues
seem to melt away without sloughing. Old ulcers,
that present reddened, glistening edges, scrofulous

Or syphilitic disease, with tumid-red, glistening swellings.

I have preferred to thus point out distinctly the indications for the use of the Rhus, without reference to the disease, according to our present nomenclature. It will be seen to point to erysipelas, typhoid fever and typhoid disease in general, and the entire list of zymotic diseases.

Our Homœopathic friends give the following indications for its use :

" Affections of the ligaments, tendons and synovial membranes ; tensions, drawing and tearing in the limbs, worse during rest, and in the cold season, or at night, in bed, frequently attended with numbness of the affected part after moving it ; creeping pains ; sensation in inner organs as if something would be torn loose ; lameness and paralysis, also hemiplegia ; vesicular erysipelas ; rhagades ; pustules which break and discharge a fluid ; hangnails ; red, shining swelling ; violent and spasmodic yawning ; evening fever, with diarrhœa ; sweat during the pains, frequently with violent trembling ; illusions of the fancy, and delirium ; pain as if the brain would be torn ; painful creeping in the head ; swelling of the head ; phagedenic scald-head ; small, soft tumors on the hairy scalp ; swelling and inflammation of the parotid glands ; acne rosacea around the mouth and chin ; nightly discharge of yellowish, or bloody saliva ; ulcerative pain in the pit of the stomach as if something would be torn off, especially when stooping or making a false step; the small of the back feels as if bruised, especially when lying still on it."

ROBINIA PSEUDO-ACACIA.
(BLACK LOCUST.)

Preparation.—Prepare a tincture from the fresh inner bark of the Black Locust, ℥viij. to Alcohol 76° Oj. Dose from gtts. j. to gtts. x.

This remedy has been but little used, yet its activity is such that we may reasonably expect that experiment will develop some valuable medicinal use. It acts on the stomach and bowels in large doses, and exerts an influence upon the nervous system. Will some of our readers test it and report?

RUMEX ACETOSELLA.
(SHEEP SORREL.)

Preparation.—Prepare a tincture from the fresh sorrel, ℥viij. to Alcohol 50° Oj. Dose, from gtts. x. to ʒss. It is employed locally in the treatment of cancer, the following formula being employed:

" *Cancer Balsam.*—Take the common Sheep Sorrel when in bloom, bruise well in a mortar, and add a small quantity of water; then press the weed so as to obtain all the juice, strain it and place in the sunshine in a pewter dish, and let it evaporate to the consistence of honey. It is then ready for use, and should be put up in sealed boxes or closely stopped bottles, in order to prevent evaporation."

A tincture of the Sorrel has a very decided action

in those cases where there is a tendency to degeneration of tissue. It makes no difference whether it is called syphilis, scrofula, or cancer, the indication for use is the replacement of tissue with lower organizations. To what extent it opposes the process of degeneration we are unable to say, the use has been so limited, but it deserves a thorough investigation. It influences the secretion of urine and urinary apparatus, but its medicinal action in this respect has yet to be determined.

Its use in the treatment of cancer has been quite extensive, and if we can believe the reports given, it has proven fully as successful as any other remedy. A full description of this method of treatment will be found in the Eclectic Journal for May, 1870, page 142.

RUMEX CRISPUS.
(YELLOW DOCK.)

Preparation.—Prepare a tincture from the fresh root, ℥viij. to Alcohol 76° Oj. Dose gtts. x. to ℈j.

We employ Rumex in cases of *bad blood* with disease of the skin; in these cases it is certainly one of the most valuable alteratives we have. In these cases we not only use it internally, but as a local application. In scrofulous disease, with deposit in glands and cellular tissue, with tendency to break down and feeble repair, I think the Rumex unequaled; here also, we use it internally and locally.

Dr. Hale reports cases of dyspepsia, with sensations of fullness and pressure in pit of stomach, pain in the chest, etc., cured by Rumex. Dr. Dunham employed it in catarrhal affections of the larynx, trachea and bronchia with advantage. I have used it in chronic sore throat with free secretion, and in broncorrhœa with good results.

The general action of the remedy is to increase waste and improve nutrition.

RUTA GRAVEOLENS.
(RUE.)

Preparation.—Prepare a tincture from the fresh plant, ℥viij. to Alcohol 76° Oj.   Dose gtts. j. to gtts. x., largely diluted with water.

Though little used, this remedy will be found to possess valuable medicinal properties. It exerts a direct influence upon the nervous system, relieving irritation and pain, and in small doses, continued, improving nutrition of the nerve centers. It acts upon the urinary and reproductive apparatus, and has been employed with advantage as a stimulant to them. In large doses, it is capable of exciting menorrhagia, inflammation, and miscarriage. The Homœopaths claim that it is a remedy " in eructations of hysteric females; prolapsus of the rectum, at every alvine evacuation ; frequent urging to urinate, with scanty emission, also of green urine, or with renewed ineffectual urging after micturition ; gravel ; miscarriage ; sterility ; corrosive leucorrhœa after suppression of the menses."

SABBATIA ANGULARIS.
(AMERICAN CENTAURY.)

Preparation.—Prepare a tincture from the fresh herb ℥viij. to Alcohol 76° Oj. Dose, gtts. j. to gtts. xx.

The Sabbatia has had a considerable reputation as a prophylactic against periodic diseases, and in their treatment—it would be well to thoroughly investigate this action. As a bitter tonic, it may be successfully employed in atonic states of the intestinal canal with increased mucous secretion. Probably it will prove useful in all diseases of mucous membranes, where there is profuse secretion. It has been but little used of late, but it deserves study.

SALIX NIGRA.
(BLACK WILLOW).

Preparation.—Prepare a tincture from the recent bark, ℥viij. to Alcohol 50° Oj. Dose from gtts. v. to ℥j.

Whilst this, as well as other varieties of the willow, possess feeble tonic and antiperiodic properties, there are so many better remedies of this class that it would be well to dispense with its use altogether, had it no other action. But there is a class of cases in which the Salix is a very decided antiperiodic, and if these can be distinguished, the remedy will be valuable. I believe it is in those in which there is increased secretion from mucous membranes, and especially where there is the septic tendency, marked by fetid discharges, foul tongue, etc. In typhoid disease it may be employed both as a tonic and antiseptic, using the smaller dose named. The remedy is easily prepared, and may well replace some inferior articles that have hitherto been employed.

SALVIA OFFICINALIS.
(SAGE.)

Preparation.—Prepare a tincture from the fresh plant when in flower 3viij. to Alcohol 76° Oj. Dose from gtts. j. to gtts. xx.

The Sage exerts a specific tonic influence on the skin, and to a less extent upon the kidneys and mucous membranes. It is not an active remedy, and hence too much must not be expected from it. We employ it where the skin is soft and relaxed, with an enfeebled circulation and cold extremities. In the treatment of colliquative perspiration it answers an excellent purpose, if the condition above is maintained. If, however, the night sweat is preceded with hectic fever, and a dry, harsh skin, it will be useless.

It will prove a good remedy in increased secretion of urine of low specific gravity; in such cases it may be associated with Belladonna. It may also be associated with the bitter tonics in all cases in which there is atony and increased secretion from mucous membranes.

SAMBUCUS CANADENSIS.
(Elder.)

Preparation.—Prepare a tincture from the fresh inner bark of the Elder, ℥viij. to Alcohol 50° Oj. Dose gtts. ij. to gtts. x.

The Elder is a stimulant to all the excretory organs increasing secretion. It may be employed for the general purposes of an alterative—increasing waste, in syphilis, scrofula, and other diseases attended by deposits or depravation of tissues. It is especially useful in these cases where there is an œdematous condition, or fullness of tissue from an increased amount of water. We meet a case of chronic disease occasionally, in which the tissues are full and flabby, evidently from too much water; in these Sambucus is a good remedy. It may be employed in dropsy, though its action is not so decided as the Apocynum.

As a local application the Sambucus is specific to those eruptions that arise on full tissues (as above), and are attended with abundant serous discharge. Thus in some forms of eczema, especially eczema infantilis or *milk scall*, and in the above form of the disease, it will alone effect a cure. We also employ it in indolent ulcers, with soft œdematous borders, and serous secretion, and in mucous patches with free secretion. An ointment is prepared by simmering the inner bark in fresh butter (old style), or a glycerole may be made, with the addition of the usual quantity of starch.

20

SANGUINARIA CANADENSIS.
(BLOOD ROOT.)

Preparation.—Prepare a tincture from the recent dried root, ℥viij. to Alcohol 76° Oj. Dose from a fraction of a drop to five drops. Nitrate of Sanguinarina is a valuable preparation, and may be dispensed in syrup, in the proportion of grs. ij. to ℥j. Dose, gtts. x. to ℥j.

In full doses we employ the Sanguinaria as a stimulant to mucous membranes. This use is valuable in bronchitis with increased secretion, and in atonic conditions of stomach and bowels with increased secretion of mucus. In minute doses we employ it in cases of cough with dryness of the throat and air passages, feeling of constriction in the chest, difficult and asthmatic breathing, with sensation of pressure. In the same doses it is a stimulant to the vegetative system of nerves, and under its use there is an improvement in the circulation, in nutrition, and secretion.

As a remedy in diseases of the respiratory tract, I prefer the Nitrate of Sanguinarina to the tincture.

SANICULA MARILANDICA.
(SANICLE.)

Preparation.—Prepare a tincture from the recent root in the proportion of ℥viij. to Alcohol 76° Oj. Dose from gtts. ij. to gtts. xx.

The Sanicula has had considerable reputation as a domestic remedy, and like most of them it has been employed for very different purposes. It evidently exerts a direct influence upon the nervous system, relieving irritation, and this probably extends to the sympathetic. It would be well to give it a trial in those cases in which there is enfeebled function with nervous irritability.

SARRACENIA PURPUREA.
(SARRACENIA.)

Preparation.—Prepare a tincture from the fresh root, in the proportion of ℥viij. to Alcohol 76° Oj. Dose from gtts. j. to gtts xx.

The experiments of Dr. Porcher, of South Carolina, showed that it exerted a marked influence on the sympathetic. From a large dose there was congestion of the head, with irregularity of the heart's action, lasting several days. Following this first effect, the general vigor of the digestive apparatus was increased, and the appetite was unusually active. It is claimed that it has been successfully employed in chlorosis, and other diseases of a similar character.

It was introduced to the notice of the profession by Dr. W. Morris, of Halifax, in 1861, as an antidote to the virus of smallpox. He made the following statements in a letter to the *American Medical Times:*

"Sir—You have by this time, in all probability, heard something of an extraordinary discovery for the cure of smallpox, by the use of 'Sarracenia Purpurea,' or Indian cup, a native plant of Nova

Scotia. I would beg of you, however, to give full
publicity to the astonishing fact, that this same
humble bog-plant of Nova Scotia is the remedy for
smallpox, in all its forms, in twelve hours after the
patient has taken the medicine. It is also as curious
as it is wonderful that, however alarming and
numerous the eruptions, or confluent and frightful
they may be, the peculiar action of the medicine is
such that very seldom is a scar left to tell the story
of the disease. I will not enter upon a physiological analysis now; it will be sufficient for my purpose to state, that it cures the disease as no other
medicine does—not by stimulating functional re-
agency, but by actual contact with the virus in the
blood, rendering it inert and harmless; and this I
gather from the fact that if either the vaccine or
variolous matter be washed with the infusion of
the Sarracenia, they are deprived of their contagious properties. The medicine, at the same time,
is so mild to the taste, that it may be mixed largely
with tea or coffee, as I have done, and given to
connoisseurs in these beverages to drink, without
their being aware of the admixture. Strange, however, to say, it is scarcely two years since science
and the medical world were utterly ignorant of this
great boon of Providence; and it would be dishon-
orable in me not to acknowledge that had it not
been for the discretion of Mr. John Thomas Lane,
of Lanespark, County Tipperary, Ireland, late of
Her Majesty's Imperial Customs of Nova Scotia, to
whom the Mec-Mac Indians had given the plant,

the world would not now be in possession of the secret. No medical man before me had ever put this medicine upon trial, but in 1861, when the whole Province of Nova Scotia was in a panic, and patients were dying at the rate of twelve and a half per cent., from May to August, Mr. Lane, in the month of May, placed the 'Sarracenia' in my hands to decide upon its merits; and, after my trials then and since, I have been convinced of its astonishing efficacy. The only functional influence it seems to have, is in promoting the flow of urine, which soon becomes limpid and abundant, and this is owing perhaps to the defecated poison or changed virus of the disease exclusively escaping through that channel. The 'Sarracenia,' I have reason to believe a powerful antidote for all contagious diseases, lepra, measles, varicella, plague, contagious typhus, and even syphilis, also a remedy in jaundice. I am strongly inclined to think it will one day play an important part in all these."

This report was confirmed by Dr. Herbert Miles, of the British Army, and Captain Hardy of the Royal Artillery. The evidence in its favor from physicians and residents of Nova Scotia would seem to be complete, that the Sarracenia has a direct prophylactic influence, and a direct and prompt curative action when the disease is developed.

The remedy, however, has been thoroughly tried by a number of physicians in the United States, and by physicians in private practice, and in the hospitals in England, with the report that if not entirely inert, it has no such antidotal power as has been ascribed to it. The evidence against it is just as positive as that in its favor.

What conclusion can we come to then? The only way we can reconcile these opposing statements is, that the same agent was not employed in both cases. In Nova Scotia, where the plant is abundant, we may suppose it was used fresh; in the United States and in England, it was dried and so old that it had lost its medical properties. I am confirmed in this opinion by my experience. Wishing to try this remedy, I obtained three samples, and neither of these possessed in the least degree the physical properties attributed to Sarracenia. When fresh, it is *bitter* and *astringent*, leaving a somewhat pungent impression on the fauces. The specimens I obtained had no taste.

In order to give the remedy a fair trial, let us have it prepared from the fresh root, obtained at the proper season. If an antidote to smallpox, its value can not be over-estimated; if it only exerts the influence over the sympathetic first named, it will prove a valuable remedy.

SCUTELLARIA LATERIFLORA.
(SKULLCAP.)

Preparation.—Prepare a tincture from the fresh herb, gathered whilst in flower, ℥viij. to Alcohol 76° Oj. Dose, from gtt. j. to gtts. xx.

. We have here another remedy that loses its medical properties by drying, until by age they are entirely dissipated. I have seen specimens furnished physicians by the drug trade that were wholly worthless—no wonder they were disappointed in its action. .

The Scutellaria exerts a direct influence upon the cerebro-spinal centers, controlling irritation. It is possible that it may also exert a tonic influence, favoring nutrition. It has been employed with success in chorea, convulsions, epilepsy, mania, etc., and especially in hysteria, monomania, and that undefined condition that we call "nervousness." I value the remedy highly, but only recommend it when prepared from the fresh plant as above.

SECALE CORNUTUM.
(ERGOT.)

Preparation. — Prepare a tincture from recent Ergot ℥viij. to Alcohol 50° Oj. Dose from the fraction of a drop to ℨj. (Ergot loses its properties with age, and it is essential, if we wish its specific action, that the tincture be prepared from the grains of the present season.)

The Ergot may be taken as the type of a specific medicine. Its action on the uterus, when fresh and good is so certain and decided, that no one can fail to see that at least one remedy acts directly. It is true, that there have been many failures in obtaining this action, but this can be attributed to worthless medicine; a large amount of that furnished physicians from drug-houses being inert from age.

Ergot may be employed in two ways, to facilitate labor. In quite small doses, say—℞ Tincture of Ergot, ʒj.; Water, ʒij.; a teaspoonful every half hour or hour, it exerts a stimulant influence, strengthening uterine contractions, and aiding dilatation of the os. It is especially useful in those cases in which there is a feeble circulation, with puffiness of face, and œdema of the feet—among the worst cases we are called to treat. Associated with small doses of Lobelia, it is an admirable remedy in rigidity, the os being thick and doughy. Its common use in large doses, in the second stage of labor, is so well known that it need not be described.

We employ Ergot in small doses, in the latter months of gestation, when there are false pains, with weight and pressure in the pelvis, fullness of labia with uneasiness, œdema, and especially if there is dullness and hebetude, with tendency to coma. In these cases no remedy will give greater satisfaction.

Ergot is a spinal stimulant, and influences the vegetative system of nerves. In some respects its action is similar to Belladonna, especially upon the circulation. Not unfrequently, we find it necessary to alternate them in order to maintain this influence.

In any case, marked by an enfeebled capillary circulation, with tendency to congestion, especially of the nervous centers, Ergot may be prescribed with advantage.

This stimulant influence upon the spinal-cord and sympathetic is manifested in contraction of non-striated muscular fiber. Hence Ergot becomes an important remedy in hemorrhage when dependent upon atony.

SCILLA MARITIMA.
(SQUILL.)

Preparation. — Prepare a tincture from the bulb ʒviij. to Alcohol 50° Oj. Dose from gtt. j. to gtts. x.

In the larger dose, the Squill is a stimulant to mucous membranes, especially those of the air passages, and may be employed to check profuse secretion. In minute doses it relieves irritation of mucous tissues and stimulates secretion.

In dropsy, presenting a dry, harsh skin, parched tongue, fevered lips, and contraction of features, the Squill may be employed as a diuretic. In the majority of cases it has been used with Digitalis, the dose being large, but it then proved beneficial in the opposite class of cases—where the circulation was feeble.

Though it has been so extensively employed, it needs to be re-studied.

SCROPHULARIA MARILANDICA.
(FIGWORT.)

Preparation.—Prepare a tincture from the leaves and root, ʒviij. to Alcohol 76° Oj. Dose from gtts. v. to gtts. xx.

21

The Scrophularia stimulates waste and excretion, and is probably as certain in its action as any of our vegetable alteratives. Beyond this it seems to exert a marked influence in promoting the removal of cacoplastic deposits. We employ it in scrofula, in secondary syphilis, in chronic inflammation with exudation of material of low vitality, and in chronic skin diseases. In the latter case it is frequently used as a local application, as well as an internal remedy.

It exerts an influence upon the urinary and reproductive organs, and has been employed in some obscure affections of these with advantage. Still it is feeble and slow, and too much must not be expected from it.

SENECIO AUREUS.
(LIFE ROOT.)

Preparation.—Prepare a tincture from the fresh herb and root, ℥viij. to Alcohol 76° Oj. Dose from gtt. j. to gtts. x. (Much disappointment has been experienced from the purchase of the crude article when old, and from worthless preparations. I would advise the practitioner, when it can be obtained, to prepare his own tincture from the fresh plant.)

The Senecio exerts a specific influence upon the reproductive organs of the female, and to a less extent upon the male. It relieves irritation and strengthens functional activity. Hence it has acquired the reputation of a " uterine tonic." It may be prescribed in all cases in which there is an atonic condition of ovaries or uterus, with derangement of function. It makes little difference whether it is amenorrhœa, dysmenorrhœa or menorrhagia, or whether it takes the form of increased mucous or purulent secretion, or displacement. The remedy acts slowly, and sufficient time must be given.

In the male we prescribe it in cases of fullness and weight in the perineum, dragging sensations in the testicle, and difficult or tardy urination. In both male and female we sometimes use it with advantage in painful micturition with tenesmus.

SILPHIUM PERFOLIATUM.
(INDIAN CUP-PLANT)

Preparation.—Prepare a tincture from the fresh root, ℥viij. to Alcohol 76° Oj. Dose from gtt. j. to gtts. x. in water.

The action of this variety of Silphium, if we are to believe the reports of the few who use it, is very direct and certain upon the chylopoietic viscera. It is claimed that it is one of the best remedies in the treatment of ague-cake, and congestion of liver and spleen, so frequently associated with chronic intermittents. It is but little employed, but deserves thorough investigation.

SILPHIUM GUMMNIFERUM.
(Rosin Weed.)

Preparation.—Prepare a tincture from the fresh plant, ℥viij. to Alcohol 76° Oj. Dose, from gtt. j. to gtts. x. The tincture of the root may be employed in some cases of cough, but is not so good as from the plant.

The Rosin Weed exerts a direct influence upon the respiratory tract, especially upon the nerve centers controlling the function. Its principal use thus far has been in the treatment of asthma, in some cases of which its action has been very decided. I think the cases in which it has proven most beneficial, are those in which there is a spasmodic dry cough, with sensations of dryness and constriction in the throat. I have not found it beneficial in lymphatic persons, or where there was congestion of mucous membranes, or profuse secretion.

I have employed it in the treatment of cough, with some advantage, but can not specify the cases in which it was useful or those in which it failed. It deserves thorough investigation, and will probably prove a valuable remedy. The tincture of the root has been furnished the profession by druggists, and the want of success with it is no evidence that the preparation from the plant is not anti-asthmatic.

SODÆ HYPOSULPHIS.
(HYPOSULPHITE OF SODA.)

SODÆ SULPHIS.
(SULPHITE OF SODA.)

It is well to procure these salts of reliable manufacturers (say Powers & Weightman), as there are many imperfect specimens in the market. The first is in the form of large colorless transparent crystals, freely soluble in water, the second in white prismatic crystals soluble in four parts of cold water: a want of solubility should cause the preparation to be rejected. It should be kept tightly corked, for it changes by exposure to the air. Dose, grs. x. to grs. xxx. every two or three hours.

In the first part of this work (Alkalies), will be found the general indication for the use of alkaline salts. They are very distinct, and can not be mistaken—pallid mucous membranes, and white coating on the tongue.

We employ the Sulphite and Hyposulphite of Soda as antizymotics, where there are the indications for the use of an alkaline salt as above. As a general rule, the indications for these salts will be—pallidity of mucous membranes, with a thick, pasty, white or dirty-white fur upon the tongue.

The influence of zymotic causes of disease on the fluids and solids is not well understood, but we know that it impairs their life, even if it does not cause more rapid sepsis. In some cases this im-

pairment of vital power is all the change that can
be noted, retrograde metamorphosis progressing
more slowly than in health or ordinary disease.
But the remedies we are studying are more than
antiseptics — they antagonize the zymotic cause
whether it produces sepsis or not.

In local diseases from a zymotic cause, as diphtheria, cynanche maligna, some forms of catarrh
and influenza, erysipelas, surgical fever, etc., these
remedies exert their specific action when locally
employed, as well as in their internal administration. The indications, however, must be as named
above—pallidity, with pasty exudates upon tongue.

Their action in arresting the growth of microscopic fungi, and during diseases arising from this
cause, is specific. In yeasty vomiting, presenting
sarcina ventriculi, the disease is speedily checked
by the Sulphites. In some forms of apthous sore
mouth and throat, speedy relief is given by their
local application. Some chronic skin diseases are
rendered very stubborn by these minute growths,
and here also the Sulphites will prove valuable.

SULPHUROUS ACID.

We consider the Sulphurous Acid here, rather
than under the head of Acids, from its relations to
the Sulphites just noticed. We employ it as an
anti-zymotic, and a parasiticide, and not for the
common purposes of an acid, though here, as in the
uses of the Alkaline Sulphites, there must be the

general indications for an acid, as there was with them for an alkali.

The Sulphurous Acid, like the Alkaline Sulphites, specifically antagonizes zymotic causes of disease. It is well to keep in mind the fact that this is something more than simply arresting or modifying the septic process, for we have already seen that the zymotic influence frequently destroys the life of the fluids and solids without producing putrescency.

We prescribe Sulphurous Acid as an anti-zymotic in those cases which present reddened mucous membranes, with brownish coatings of tongue and sordes. Given, the indications for the use of an anti-zymotic, with the indications for the use of an acid, we select the Sulphurous Acid.

Sulphurous Acid may be employed in yeasty vomiting, in apthous mouth and throat, or wherever the presence of microscopic fungi is suspected, with the same certainty as the Sulphite of Soda. We also use it in porrigo, trichosis of scalp, ptyriasis versicolor, with excellent results. As a local application it should be diluted with from two to six parts of water.

I wish to call especial attention to its use in some diseases of the throat, by the spray or atomizing apparatus. In diphtheria, with dark redness of mucous membranes, and fullness with relaxation, there is no local remedy equal to Sulphurous Acid spray. It is equally beneficial in those cases of cynanche maligna, with dark redness of mucous membranes. Whilst in ordinary sore throat from cold, with dusky discoloration, it offers one of the best local applications in the Materia Medica.

SOLANUM DULCAMARA.
(BITTERSWEET).

Preparation.—Prepare a tincture from the fresh twigs gathered in the fall, when the leaves have fallen, ℥viij. to Alcohol 70° Oj. Dose, from gtt. j. to gtts. x.

The Bittersweet has the reputation of being a good alterative, in cutaneous diseases, syphilis, scrofula and inflammatory deposits, and we conclude that it increases waste and excretion. It exerts a marked influence upon the cerebro-spinal centers, when used in large doses, but this has not been studied.

I would advise the employment of the remedy in small doses in those cases of chronic disease in which the circulation is feeble, the hands and feet cold and purplish, with fullness of tissues and tendency to œdema. I do not know that it will prove better than other remedies, but it deserves investigation.

SPONGIA USTA.
(BURNT SPONGE).

Take of ordinary sponge a sufficient quantity, cut it in pieces, and burn it in a close iron vessel until it is brown and can be pulverized without much trouble. Now, take of this powder four ounces, pack in a percolator, and gradually add Alcohol 76° Oj   Dose of the tincture from the fraction of a drop to ℥ss.

I give the formula for the preparation of a tincture of burnt sponge, not because I think it possesses all the properties attributed to it by Homœopaths, but that it may be tested. I have used it in some cases with seeming advantage, and have seen results following its prescription by others, that in the ordinary use of medicine we would call remarkable cures. A quotation from Jahr's Repertory will show the Homœopathic uses:

" Diseases of the lymphatic vessels and glands; heat, with dry, hot skin, thirst, headache and delirium; redness of the eyes, with burning and lachrymation; frequent eructations, with cutting and tearing in the stomach; relaxed feeling in the stomach, as if the stomach were open; orchitis; induration of the testes; pain in the larynx on touching it and turning the head; *burning in the larynx and trachea; dryness, husky and hoarse voice; inflammation of the larynx, trachea and bronchi; croup; laryngeal and tracheal phthisis;* cough, deep from the chest, with soreness and burning, or chronic cough with yellowish expectoration and hoarseness; wheezing inspirations; asthma with amenorrhœa; goitre; hard goitre.'

STAPHYLEA TRIFOLIA.
(BLADDER NUT.)

Preparation.—Prepare a tincture from the bark of the root, ℥viij. to Alcohol 76° Oj. Dose from gtts. v. to ℨj.

The Staphylea has been confounded with the Ptelea, until we hardly know whether a writer in the olden times was describing one or the other. The probabilities are, however, that the article described by Prof. I. G. Jones, and valued so highly by him as a tonic, was the article under consideration. At least it would be well for some of our friends who know the article, to procure specimens and thoroughly test it.

Dr. Jones claimed that it was a pure unirritating tonic, having a soothing influence upon mucous membranes. He employed it in the convalescence from fevers and inflammations, and whenever the stomach was feeble and irritable.

STILLINGIA SYLVATICA.
(STILLINGIA.)

Preparation.—Prepare a tincture from the recent dried root, ℥viij. to Alcohol 98° Oj. Dose from gtt. j. to gtts x.

Stillingia increases waste and excretion, but its principal action probably is upon the lymphatic system, favoring the formation of good lymph, hence good blood and nutrition. Experience shows that it favorably influences the system in secondary syphilis, in some forms of scrofula, and in cases of chronic disease where the tissues are feeble and not readily removed and renewed.

I believe it to be more especially useful in those cases where there is predominant affection of mucous membranes, and secondly, where the skin is involved. In these cases I have used the simple tincture as above, largely diluted with water, with much better results than I have obtained from any of the compounds of Stillingia or alterative syrups. Evidently in the ordinary manufacture of "Compound Syrup of Stillingia," the virtues of Stillingia, if it has any, are wholly lost, simply because water or dilute alcohol is not a proper menstruum.

Stillingia exerts a specific influence upon the mucous membranes of the throat, larynx, and bronchii, relieving irritation and favoring normal nutrition and functional activity. Some cases of chronic pharyngitis of years' standing, have been relieved by this remedy, after other treatment had failed. It is an excellent remedy in the treatment of some cases of chronic laryngitis, speedily relieving the irritation and cough, and we also employ it in chronic bronchitis with like good results. Now if it is possible to determine the class of cases in which it is thus beneficial, the reader may use it with advantage.

So far as my experience extends, they are those with tumid, red, glistening mucous membranes, with scanty secretion. This condition indeed seems to be the index for the use of the remedy for every purpose. In syphilis, in scrofula, in chronic inflammation with deposits, the same red glistening color, with scanty secretion, is my guide to the use of Stillingia.

STRYCHNOS NUX VOMICA.
(Nux Vomica.)

Preparation. — Prepare a tincture from freshly powdered seeds, ℥viij. to Alcohol 76° Oj. Dose, from the fraction of a drop to five drops. A solution of Strychnia may be prepared after the following formula: ℞ Sulphate of Strychnia, grs. iv.; Water, ℥iv.; dose, gtts. v. $\frac{1}{98}$ gr. to gtts. xx. $\frac{1}{24}$ gr.

Nux Vomica exerts a specific influence upon the intestinal canal and associate viscera that renders it a most valuable remedy.

In minute doses we employ it to arrest nausea and vomiting, when this arises from gastric irritability and not from irritant material in the stomach. The cases are those in which there is feebleness of the organs, and not where there is irritation and inflammation. For this purpose we employ it in cholera infantum with marked benefit, and in cholera morbus and Asiatic cholera to relieve this symptom.

It is *the* remedy in all cases of congestion of *liver*, spleen, or portal circle. Given, a feeling of fullness in right hypochondrium, pain in side or shoulder, sallowness of face, yellowness of eyes, yellow coat on tongue, I prescribe Nux Vomica with a certainty that I never felt in the olden time.

If an intermittent fever presents these evidences of visceral derangement, Nux Vomica is *the* antiperiodic, or at least it prepares the way for the kindly and curative action of Quinine. In bilious remittent fevers, with these symptoms, Nux Vomica is the first remedy indicated. In diarrhœa, with these symptoms, we prescribe it with the certainty that the discharges will be speedily arrested, and the stomach and intestinal canal left in good condition. In dyspepsia, with these symptoms, we obtain speedy and permanent relief from the use of the remedy.

It is here, as we have found it in the consideration of other remedies, if you can determine the exact indication for its use, you employ it whenever you find these indications, no matter what may be the name of the disease, or the condition of the patient otherwise.

We employ it to relieve pain in the stomach and bowels, where there is atony. It makes no difference whether it is the colic of childhood or of the adult, acute or chronic. It is not a remedy for pain dependent upon irritation with determination of blood, or upon muscular spasm.

In addition to the symptoms named, as indicating the use of Nux Vomica, may be named hypochondriac pain, umbilical pain, or pain in forehead associated with nausea; yellowish or brownish maculæ, in chronic disease, are also indications for its use. In some cases, a peculiar yellowish sallow ring around the mouth, will be found indicative of impairment of innervation from the solar plexus, and Nux will prove the remedy.

We find this peculiarity in the action of Nux Vomica, which we have noticed with some of the more prominent of the specific medicines, and which, indeed, is true of all—when distinctly indicated, it may be *the* remedy for the entirety of a disease. Thus, taking a fever presenting the symptoms of nausea, hypochondriac and umbilical pains, full, moist tongue, with slight yellow coat, and sallow skin. Nux Vomica relieves gastric irritation, is prompt and sedative, relieves irritation of the nervous system, stimulates secretion — indeed it is prompt and sedative. Take a case of dysentery with these characteristic symptoms, and relief is speedy and the cure rapid.

The influence of Nux Vomica and Strychnia upon the spinal cord is well known, and this seems to be its principal use in medicine. Whilst I think it better, in the majority of cases, to restrict its use as above, there are some in which we employ it for its influence upon the nervous system alone. These are :—

In typhoid and asthenic disease, where there is impairment of spinal innervation, and in consequence imperfect or enfeebled respiration, we give Strychnia or Nux Vomica with advantage. Indeed, in those cases in which the respiratory function can only be carried on under the influence of the will, it is the only remedy we can rely on.

In the same classes of disease, the tendency to retention of urine is met by the use of the same remedy.

In some cases of the same diseases, where a feeble circulation is associated with general impairment of muscular power, and inability to co-ordinate muscular movement, we use Nux Vomica with advantage.

Nux Vomica or Strychnia should never be employed in the treatment of paralysis so long as any evidence of inflammatory action exists; neither should it be used, if there are marked evidences of cerebro-spinal congestion, until this is removed. It is the first remedy employed in cases of paralysis presenting the symptoms of visceral derangement we have already named. In other cases it is only employed as a nerve stimulant, when the nerve centers are free from disease.

SULPHUR.

Preparation.—Prepare Sulphur for dispensing, by thorough trituration with two parts of Sugar of Milk. Dose from gr. j. to ℥ss.

We employ Sulphur as a restorative in those cases in which there is a deficiency of this element in the blood. "All the protein-compounds contain Sulphur, which seems to be one of their essential constituents, not capable of entire separation without the complete destruction of the organic substance," (Carpenter). There are few, probably, who have

thought of Sulphur in this relation ; they supply
Iron as the basis of red corpuscles, Phosphorus for
the nutrition of the nervous system, but the protein
tissues must get their supply of Sulphur from the
food, or do without.

The indication for the use of Sulphur as a restorative is, enfeebled nutrition associated with de-
coloration of tissues, and secretions. The skin is
blanched, the iris loses color, the hair is lighter in
color in the young, changes rapidly to gray in the
middle aged, and the urine is light colored as is the
feces. The presence of cystine in the urine is an
indication for the administration of Sulphur.

We also employ Sulphur in those cases in which
there is excessive fetor of the excretions. We will
occasionally find a case of chronic disease, in which
the breath, the secretion from the skin, the urine,
and the feces have a peculiar cadaverous odor, and
we notice that with this there is a remarkable tendency to decomposition, and to breaking down of
tissue.

It is possible that this may be explained, by the
necessity of Sulphur in the formation of the tau-
rine of the bile. If this secretion of the liver is
the normal antiseptic, and controls putrescency in
the body, we can see why a deficiency of Sulphur
may lead to the condition above named, and its administration be directly curative.

STICTA PULMONARIA.

From this variety of Lichen, found growing on trees in many parts of the United States, is prepared a tincture in the usual manner. It is a remedy introduced by the Homœopathists, and thus far I have employed their tincture. I use it in the proportion of ℥j. to ℥ij. to water ℥iv.; a teaspoonful every three or four hours.

I have employed it with success in atonic lesions of the respiratory organs, attended with dull pains in the chest, increased by full inspiration. There is also a sense of soreness, as if bruised, or that follows very severe exertion. In these cases it exerted a marked influence, relieving the cough and unpleasant sensations; even checking the chills, hectic fever and night sweats, in confirmed phthisis, for some considerable time.

I have also used it in a few cases of rheumatism with benefit. Dr. C. C. Price of Baltimore says :— "I have used Sticta in rheumatism very extensively for the past three or four years. I find it most useful in those cases, where, in connection with the larger joints, the small ones are also involved. It matters not whether fingers or toes, there is swelling, heat, and circumscribed *redness* of the joints."

I would be very glad if some of our practitioners would test *Variolaria Faginea* (Lichen Fagineus) and the Lichen Parietina. Both have been employed successfully in the treatment of ague, and are powerful stimulants and restoratives.

22

SYMPLOCARPUS FŒTIDUS.
(SKUNK CABBAGE.)

Preparation.—Prepare a tincture from the fresh root, ʒviij. to Alcohol 76° Oj. Dose from gtt. j. to gtts. v.

Though the Skunk Cabbage has been extensively used, it has been in combination with other remedies, and the reports are so vague that we can not estimate its remedial action. It exerts a very decided influence upon the nervous system, relieving irritation and promoting normal functional activity. This, probably, will be its principal use. The remedy deserves to be thoroughly studied.

TANACETUM VULGARE.
(TANSY.)

Preparation.—Prepare a tincture from the fresh herb gathered in August, using ʒviij. to Alcohol 76° Oj. Dose gtts. j. to gtt. xx. As a local application to the throat use one part of the tincture to four to ten parts of hot water, with a spray apparatus; or not having this, vaporize the fluid and let the patient inhale the steam.

In small doses the tincture as above prepared will furnish a cheap and agreeable stomachic, relieving irritation and improving functional activity. It exerts a decided stimulant influence upon the female reproductive organs, and may be employed in functional diseases when such influence is desirable.

As a local application by spray or inhalation, it is a very valuable remedy in the treatment of diphtheria, and some forms of acute inflammation of the throat, and in epidemic catarrh. I have employed it in these cases with most marked advantage, and value it very highly.

TARAXACUM DENS LEONIS.
(Dandelion.)

Preparation.—Prepare a tincture from the fresh root gathered in July or August, ℥viij. to Alcohol 76° Oj. Dose from gtts. v. to ʒss.

The Taraxacum loses its medical properties by drying, hence that usually supplied by the drug trade is wholly inert. Prepared as above, it will prove a valuable remedy.

It exerts a stimulant influence upon the entire gastro-intestinal tract, promoting functional activity. Whilst its action is feeble, it is very certain, and will frequently prove more desirable than the more active remedies.

TELA ARANEÆ.
(Spider's Web.)

From the web of the common house spider, prepare a tincture by macerating ℥ij. in Alcohol 98° Oj. for ten days. Dose, gtt. j. to gtts. x.

It is claimed to be a very certain remedy in the cure of intermittents. I give a formula for its preparation, that it may be tested. The tincture of the Aranea Diadema is employed in Germany by some Homœopaths, and cases reported in which the cure was speedy and permanent.

THUJA OCCIDENTALIS.
(ARBOR VITÆ.)

Preparation.—Prepare a tincture from the fresh leaves, ℥viij. to Alcohol 76° Oj Dose from gtt. j. to gtts. xx.

The leaves of the Arbor Vitæ has been a popular remedy in the treatment of intermittent and remittent fever, rheumatism, scurvy, etc. It would be well for some of our practitioners to prepare a tincture and test it.

TRIFOLIUM PRATENSE.
(RED CLOVER.)

Preparation.—Prepare a tincture from the recently dried blossoms of Red Clover, ℥viij. to Alcohol 50° Oj. Dose from gtt. j. to gtts. x.

The Red Clover exerts a specific influence in some cases of whooping cough, and in the cough of measles. It is not curative in all, but when it does good, the benefit is speedy and permanent. It may also be prescribed in other cases of spasmodic cough, in laryngitis, bronchitis and phthisis. We should be able to tell the exact condition where it proves beneficial, and where it fails, but thus far the use has been wholly empirical. In the further use f the remedy all the symptoms should be noted.

It has given much satisfaction thus far, and is likely to prove a very valuable remedy.

TRILLIUM PENDULUM.
(BETHROOT.)

Preparation.—Prepare a tincture from the fresh root, ℥viij. to Alcohol 76° Oj. Dose from gtt. j. to gtts. x.

The common use of Trillium in large doses obtained its astringent influence, possibly from the tannin it contains. The preparation from the fresh root named above, is but slightly astringent.

We would employ it in disease of mucous membranes with increased secretion, and expect decided benefit. In the earlier part of my practice I used Trillium in chronic bronchitis, in chronic catarrh, in cough with free expectoration, with excellent results. It needs to be thoroughly studied, and it will probably supply a want in our Materia Medica.

URTICA DIOICA.
(COMMON NETTLE.)

Preparation.—Prepare a tincture from the fresh plant, ℥viij. to Alcohol 76° Oj. Dose from gtts. j. to gtts. x.

The Urtica has been employed in some diseases of the bowels, with reported good results. An old practitioner informs me, that in chronic disease of the large intestine with increased mucous secretion, he has never found anything so beneficial as this remedy. It has also been used in diseases of the urinary organs.

It is now but little used, but deserves investigation.

VALERIANA OFFICINALIS.
(VALERIAN.)

Preparation.—Prepare a tincture from the root (as recent as can be obtained), ʒviij. to Alcohol 50° Oj. Dose from gtts. ij. to gtts. xx.

Valerian is a cerebral stimulant, and may be employed wherever a remedy of this character is indicated. It allays nervous irritability, modifies or arrests pain, promotes rest, and favors sleep, where these conditions result from an enfeebled cerebral circulation. It is very extensively used, and many times without benefit, as the condition of the nervous centers is very rarely taken into consideration.

VERATRUM VIRIDE.
(VERATRUM.)

Preparation.—Prepare a tincture from the recent root, not fully dried, ʒviij. to Alcohol 76° Oj. Dose from the fraction of a drop to three drops. Veratrum from Western New York furnishes an excellent remedy, as is that from North Carolina and Northern Georgia. Specimens I have seen from the Western States were worthless. The root should be dug in August or September, freed from dirt, and dried sufficiently to permit of shipment to the place of manufacture. Now, it should be immediately crushed, and the year's supply of tincture prepared.

As commonly prepared for the drug trade, (Norwood's excepted), it is made of the dried root kept in stock from year to year, and possesses very feeble, if any medical properties. In this case, as with some other remedies, the process of drying destroys that finer medical action upon which we depend to influence the sympathetic nervous system.

We employ the Veratrum to lessen the frequency of the heart's action. When properly used it not only lessens the frequency of the pulse, but it removes obstruction to the free circulation of the blood, and thus gives slowness, regularity, freedom, and an equal circulation in all parts of the body. This action we call arterial sedation, though the name is not a good one.

To obtain this action it is necessary that the remedy be used in small doses, frequently repeated, and that sufficient time be given to accomplish the object without disturbing function or producing depression.

Veratrum is sedative in large doses, and its influence upon the heart may be speedily obtained in this way. But in this case its influence is depressing. It evidently causes slowness of the pulse by paralyzing the cardiac nerves. If the influence is continued there is impairment of the circulation, with tendency to congestion. As a general rule, the influence of large doses can not be maintained; either the remedy produces irritation of the stomach, so that it will no longer be tolerated, or its depressing influence upon the circulation becomes so great that it must be suspended.

In small doses the Veratrum is a stimulant to all the vegetative processes. Acting through the sympathetic or ganglionic system of nerves, it removes obstruction to the capillary circulation, gives tone to the vascular system, and strength to the heart. As the obstacles to a free circulation are removed, and the vessels through which the blood is distributed and returned, regain their normal condition, there is less necessity for increased action upon the part of the heart; and as the power of the heart is increased, there is less necessity for frequent contraction.

I give this as a theory of the action of Veratrum, but whether true or not, there is no question with regard to the facts as above stated.

Veratrum is the remedy for sthenia, where there is a frequent but free circulation. It is also the remedy where there is an active capillary circulation, both in fever and inflammation. A full and bounding pulse, a full and hard pulse, and a corded or wiry pulse, if associated with inflammation of serous tissues, call for this remedy.

As was remarked when describing Aconite, the Veratrum exerts a similar influence in acute inflammation, and directly controls the inflammatory process in its first stages. As a rule, the remedies that will cure fever will cure inflammation. To this I believe there are no exceptions, if a proper diagnosis is made, and we are governed by the same indications for prescribing. Aconite, Veratrum, Gelseminum, Belladonna, Nux Vomica, Quinia, and other direct remedies, may be prescribed with the same certainty in inflammation as in fever. There is the same necessity for securing a good condition of stomach and upper intestine for digestion, and giving proper food. The same necessity for securing normal waste and excretion, and having the tissues renewed from good blood. The pallid tongue calls for alkalies, the dark redness of mucous membranes for acids, the pasty white coat for the sulphites, etc.

My experience teaches me that local inflammations are reached directly by this direct medication, and with a certainty a hundred times greater than by the old routine of internal and external counter-irritation. It makes no difference where its location, how great or how little, the treatment is exactly the same as for a fever presenting the same symptoms or indications for remedies.

It must not be expected that the indications for remedies will be as pronounced in the case of inflammation as in fever, but they are always sufficient.

I have treated inflammation of the lungs with Veratrum alone, Veratrum with Gelseminum, Veratrum with Ipecac, Ipecac alone, Aconite alone, with a success I never saw obtained from the use of nau-

23

seants and counter-irritation.   Other cases required
the use of the Sulphites, of Quinia, or the mineral
acids.   I am not alone in this experience, for scores
of our more recent students, who have learned this
practice in lectures, give testimony to its success.

The local application of Veratrum, in the early
stages of a superficial inflammation, will not unfrequently arrest its progress.   In this way we use it in
erysipelas, in phlegmonous inflammation of cellular
tissue, in felons, diseases of the bones, tonsilitis, etc.

We employ Veratrum in the treatment of chronic
disease for its stimulant influence upon the vegetative processes.   Properly used, we find that it lessens
the frequency of the pulse, giving a free and uniform circulation ; it lessens the temperature ; it increases waste and excretion ; and finally it stimulates digestion and nutrition.

My friend, Prof. Howe, regards it as one of the
most direct and certain " Alteratives " in the Materia Medica, and in this opinion he is supported by a
large number of practitioners.   If the remedy has
the action above named, we can readily see how it
favorably influences chronic disease, and how frequently it may be employed with advantage.

VERBASCUM THAPSUS.
(MULLEIN.)

Preparation.—Prepare a tincture from the fresh
tops and smaller leaves when the plant is in flower,
℥viij. to Alcohol 50° Oj. Dose from gtts. ʋ. to ℨj.

The Verbascum exerts a mild influence upon the nervous system, quieting irritation and promoting sleep. It also allays bronchial irritation, and checks cough. It is very feeble, and has but a limited use.

VIBURNUM OPULUS.
(HIGH CRANBERRY.)

Preparation.—Prepare a tincture from the recent bark, ℥viij. to Alcohol 50° Oj. Dose, from gtts. v. to gtts. xx.

The Viburnum has been employed as an anti-spasmodic with reported success, hence its name, *cramp bark*. If we are to be guided by the descriptions of our earlier practitioners, we would conclude that it exerted a direct influence in controlling spinal irritation, and spasmodic action arising from this. I have never used it, though I think it worthy a trial.

VIBURNUM PRUNIFOLIUM.
(BLACK HAW.)

Preparation.—Prepare a tincture from the recent bark of the root, ℥viij. to Alcohol 50° Oj. Dose from gtts. v. to gtts. xx.

It is claimed in the Southern States that the Viburnum is a specific against abortion. I have been told by several parties, that it was a common practice among planters to make their slaves drink an infusion of the Viburnum daily whilst pregnant, to prevent abortion from taking the Cotton-root. A physician from Texas assured me, that from an observation of fifteen years, he was confident that it exerted this influence, and that he had prescribed it in many cases without a failure.

If it exerts this influence upon the uterus, it will prove a valuable remedy, not only as anti-abortive, but in diseases of the reproductive organs.

XANTHOXYLUM FRAXINEUM.
(PRICKLY ASH.)

Preparation.—Prepare a tincture from the berries, ℥viij. to Alcohol 98° Oj. Dose from the fraction of a drop to five drops.

The Xanthoxylum has been employed as a diffusible and topical stimulant. Its general stimulant action is not very marked, and there are many other remedies preferable. But as a stimulant to mucous tissues it has no equal in the Materia Medica. Whenever it is desirable to obtain such influence, whether of the throat, the gastro-intestinal tract, the mucous membranes of the air-passages, or of the urinary organs, we are rarely disappointed in its action. Upon the throat, the stomach, and upon the intestines, it exerts a topical influence before absorption.

In small doses we occasionally employ it in chronic diseases of mucous surfaces, with good results. The cases are as above, when the mucous membranes are enfeebled and relaxed, with hypersecretion.

APPENDIX.

The study of Specific Medication is yet in its infancy, and it is impossible to present a systematic treatise on the subject. The intention of the author in first presenting this little volume to the profession, was to lay before them a concise statement of what was really known of the direct action of medicines, and to incite to a re-study of the Materia Medica. It has well served its purpose in calling attention to the subject, in causing investigation, and in pointing out the road to a better practice of medicine.

Passing through two editions, it has required some revision, and some additions. The principal work in this direction, since its first issue, has been done in the Eclectic Medical Journal, and we propose to give here the principal articles that have appeared in the past two years.

It might be better if they were rewritten and systematized, but probably they will serve the purpose well in their original form. For if there are repetitions, there is the freshness and earnestness that attaches to a first presentation of a subject; and it is sometimes well to see how a thing grows—we can better estimate its merit.

I have no apology to offer for them. They tell the story plainly and emphatically, and I have yet seen no reason to take back ought that has been written.

The Study of Specific Medication.

I admit that the study of medicine, as I would pursue it, is more difficult than the old routine, and that it also requires an exercise of brain far beyond it. But surely, if there can be certainty in diagnosis, and precision in giving remedies, it is worth all the thought which is given it.

Think for a moment of the imperfections of our present nosology. We find the most diverse conditions of disease grouped under the same name. And hence, a list of medicines, as long as the moral law, is named, with a "*may be* given in this disease with *prospect* of advantage." No effort seems to be made to determine the exact indications for any particular remedy, and no medicine is studied with reference to its direct opposition to morbid processes.

Hence flows the *shot-gun* method of prescribing, whereby the more common drugs are combined in platoons, and fired into the sick. To a lover of fun, (medical fun I mean), there is no better reading than a druggist's prescription book, if the reader has his eyes open to its absurdity. Passing by the queer combinations of remedies, ten, twenty, thirty, fifty different ingredients, (combining compounds), we have all manner of incompatible mixtures—milky, grumous, flaky, deposits, etc—all kinds of queer tastes, agreeing only in being nasty—all kinds of activities represented in the same bottle—stimulant, sedative, narcotic, tonic, emetic, cathartic, etc. But beyond this we find the doctor ignoring the law of medicinal incompatibles, and combining his remedies so that one neutralizes the other—as giving Belladonna and Gelseminum, Belladonna and Opium, Stramonium and Opium as a local application, etc.

Read your Materia Medica, and you find the description of a remedy commencing—"this agent is *said to be* emetic, cathartic, diaphoretic, diuretic, stimulant, tonic," etc. We never get farther than a "said to be," and a "prospect of advantage." This and-so-forth that is affixed to the end of the sentence really covers what we want to know, and I have often thought that a system of rational medicine might be written under the title—"The Mysteries of And-so-forth Revealed."

I name these things, not that I want to ridicule the old methods, but that our readers may see their absurdity as I see it. I do not want to be understood as saying that all practice but mine is absurd, for I know that the large majority of physicians do prescribe in part *directly*, and do expect a definite result by so doing. And I claim further, that every physician, no matter what school of medicine he belongs to, finds success in so doing. Examine your methods of treating disease, and the remedies you use, and you can not but be convinced of the truth of this. If this is so, hold fast to all your direct remedies and increase the list as far as you can, but discard at once and forever all those shot-gun formulæ, and all indirect methods.

Need I say again "that the earlier Eclectics prescribed directly," and used "Specifics," and had success by so doing. If any one doubts it, I will be glad to have him read the five volumes of "The Medical Reformer," and the early volumes of the Eclectic Medical Journal. And get especially the early history of our indigenous remedies, and you will find that they were given *singly*, and for their *direct* curative influence.

And now we come to the really important point, how will we study Specific Medication? The question is asked me every day, and needs an answer.

As has been stated, we must study diagnosis with reference to conditions of disease, and not to select a name from the nosological list. As we must have a standard of health to start from, and as a basis of comparison, we want a thorough knowledge of physiology, and to the busy practitioner I recommend Huxley's, because it is concise and in small compass. Follow this with the "Principles of of Medicine," and we learn the physiology of disease—pathology; not with reference to an arbitrary nomenclature, but as parts of *t* diseased life. We never forget that we are dealing with *living* men, and that this which we call disease, is simply abnormal *life*.

Then comes the study of remedies with reference to their power of opposing processes of disease, and favoring the restoration of normal life. We never forget that in disease the power of living is enfeebled. We never forget that the *forces* of life are weakened, and that the tissues of the body have lost their functional power, to some degree, as well as their power of reproduction by which the life of man is continued.

We never forget that our power, however skillful we may be, is limited. We can not give life to inorganic matter, we can not grow a single hair or a cell; all that we can do is to guide and regulate the forces of life, and even this has its limits.

But whilst we want to know that our field of action is thus limited, we also wish to know that inside these limits there is a broad field for study and use to man. We learn first—not to take life; we learn secondly—how we may best conserve it, and influence its forces to an orderly activity.

As we go on in this course of study the subject becomes plainer step by step. As we cease to study *dissimilars* in the old nosology, we learn to study *similars* in specific diagnosis and medication. We learn to know that similar conditions of disease are always treated alike, no matter what the technical name of the disease, or its location. And as we thus always prescribe for pathological conditions, we find at last that the practice of medicine is really simplified, and it becomes a pleasure, instead of being laborious and unpleasant from its uncertainty.—*E. M. Journal, March*, 1872.

Some Phases of Specific Medication.

The basis of specific medication is specific diagnosis. If the physician can not determine the *exact* pathological conditions, his prescription must be *inexact*, and in proportion as it is so—uncertain.

Is it not the fact, that the common idea of the " uncertainty of medicine " leads to superficial study, carelessness in examination, careless prescribing, to downright quackery?

Train a man in the popular belief of idiosyncrasies, inscrutable providences, *et id omne*, and why should he give much thought to the study of disease. This prescribing for the sick is a random business at best, and he fires his Materia Medica at his patients, expecting by some lucky shot to hit the disease; if he should happen to knock the patient into the next world—is there not an inscrutable Providence?

But the physician need not fire wholly at random, he may fire in platoons—fire and fall back. For instance, in all diseases, excepting those attended with diarrhœa, he may fire the class cathartics at his patient, and continue so long as the patient has bowels to respond. He will find on turning to his text-books, a mass of authority to sustain him in this course, much further indeed than he dare go. Or he may charge his patient with emetics, supplement these with diaphoretics and diuretics, with a skirmish line of Quinine and Opium. Or he may make a hodge-podge of them all—a grand *corps de battaile*—and assault the enemy flank and rear.

Of course the patient has no need of stomach and bowels for the digestion of food whilst sick. As he *is* sick, the unpleasant sensations that attend and follow such giving of medicine, need not be taken into account. As there *is* disturbance of all the vegetative and vital functions in disease, the additional disturbance by medicine is a matter of small moment. Why should we bother our heads about such small matters as these? Have we not the testimony of ages of *authority*—that "this is the way, the truth and the life?"

And is it not much easier to walk in the way of our fathers?

But it is not of random medication that we want to talk, further than to adorn our moral and point this tale. The absurdities of old physic are patent to all, a matter of every-day experience; we want to learn a better way, if there is one.

The *first phase* of Specific Medication is so plain, " that he who runs may read;" it appeals directly to every man's experience and better judgment; and it needs but a clear presentation to obtain the assent of every man, not governed by prejudice. We might state it as follows:

There is a standard of healthy life. Disease is a *departure* from it. The province of rational medicine is to restore it. This unit of life that constitutes a living man is clearly divisible, and is divided by physiologists into several parts, which may be studied separately, and for each of which we have a standard of healthy life. Thus, we study the circulation of the blood, respiration, digestion and blood-making, nutrition, waste and excretion, as well as the structure of the blood, and the solids, and the essential conditions of life—heat and electricity. And as we study these separately in health, that we may fix in our mind a healthy standard of life, so we study them separately in disease that we may know its exact character.

We see that the departure from health must be in one of three directions—above, below, from— or according to the classification of Dr. Williams, " in excess, defect, perversion." Common sense would at once suggest a rational treatment—if there is an excess of function, bring it down to the normal standard—if there is a defect, bring it up—if there is a perversion, correct it—always selecting remedies that influence the part or function affected, directly.

The first lesson in specific diagnosis is to recognize the separate lesions which compose a disease, and classify them as named above. We say, that at once a rational treatment is suggested, but this is only so, to one who has given the subject some thought; the old therapeutics shed but little light upon it.

The first lesson in specific therapeutics is, to learn that remedies are selective, and that when introduced into the circulation through the stomach, they specially influence certain parts and functions, and that this action is unvarying.

Now, it is but a simple application of common sense to say, that if we desire to influence the circulation of the blood, we shall select a remedy that acts upon the circulatory system, and not one that acts upon the bowels, skin, kidneys, brain, or other parts. And it is only one step farther to say, that the remedy should be selected with regard to the character of the lesion—if in excess, that it will bring it down—if defective, that it will bring it up—if perverted, that it will correct it.

This, the reader will see, is but the application of logic to the practice of medicine. We want precision of observation, and thus applying the unvarying rules of logic, we reason to correct conclusions; and a practice thus based must be right. You can't call this theorizing—it is plain matter-of-fact—clearly demonstrable in its premises and conclusions—and as absolutely true at the bedside as in the lecture-room.

The second lesson in specific diagnosis is, to determine the relative importance of these lesions. We want to know which stands first, and serves as a basis—we might properly call this the *basic lesion*—and then the relative importance of others which have grown upon it. When we come to study the "second phase" of specific medication we will find this to be a principal feature.

We can best illustrate this lesson, by reference to cases :— For instance, many simple fevers and inflammations have as a basic lesion, the disturbance of the circulation, and the increase of temperature; arrest of secretion, loss of appetite, digestion and nutrition, depravation of the blood, and derangement of innervation, are based upon them. The disease may really *be* a very active and severe one, and yet rest so wholly upon the lesion of circulation, that if this is corrected, they all fade away, and the patient rapidly convalesces. The special sedative, associated with the proper bath, becomes in these cases absolutely curative, and no other medicine is necessary.

But again, we find cases in which the lesions of circulation and temperature are quite as marked, and yet the sedative is not curative; in some cases, indeed, it is not sedative even. Let us take two very common cases illustrative of this:

A typical malarial fever gives us quite as frequent a pulse and exalted a temperature, as in the case where the sedative alone was curative—but now we find it only preparative—the lesion of the blood is the *basic* lesion. We prepare the patient for the use of Quinine, or in some cases give it alone, and the Quinine is curative.

Again, a patient is suffering with acute fever or inflammation, the pulse quite as frequent, the temperature as high, and yet the sedative has no more influence than so much water, unless it be to irritate the stomach. What now? A direct sedative *not* influencing the circulation—have we here an idiosyncrasy? Oh, no! not at all! the only trouble is, that the lesion of the circulation and temperature is not the *basic* lesion. Supposing we examine the tongue and find it *pallid* with *white* coat, we say at once here is a lesion of the blood, a salt of soda is required. We give it, and now the sedative acts kindly, or indeed it may not be necessary, simple bicarbonate of soda lessening the frequency of the pulse more markedly than Veratrum.

We find the same is the case where the symptoms point to the Alkaline Sulphites, Muriatic Acid, Sulphurous Acid, Chlorate of Potash, Phosphorus, Iron, Copper, or even Cod Oil, or food.

If for instance, in an endemic of typhoid fever, we find *deep redness* of mucous membranes, this being characteristic of the *basic* lesion—a *want of acid*—we find that Muriatic Acid becomes sedative, stimulant, restorative, increases secretion, checks diarrhœa, stops delirium, indeed does all for the patient that we can wish. Most times we supplement it with other remedies acting in these directions—but occasionally it is safest to trust to the acid alone.

I have obtained quite as marked results from the use of Sulphurous Acid in the treatment of typho-malarial fever this year, as I have in the use of Sulphite of Soda in other seasons.

Again, we find cases where the predominant affection is of the nervous system. For instance, the face is flushed, eyes bright, pupils contracted, increased heat of scalp, restless and sleepless, determination of blood to the brain—Gelseminum becomes our best sedative. Why? Because it quiets the irritation of the brain, and removes, this, which is the *basic* lesion.

So it is in the opposite condition—enfeebled capillary circulation, and tendency to congestion of the cerebro-spinal centers. The pulse may be quite as frequent, the temperature as high, secretions arrested, blood poisoning rapid, and yet sedatives are not sedative. Why? Because there is an underlying lesion. We must influence the vegetative system of nerves first, to restore capillary circulation—and then our other remedies act kindly. I have sat by the bedside and seen the pulse fall from 140 beats per minute to 100, and the temperature from 107° to 101°, in four hours, under the influence of Belladonna alone—and yet Belladonna is *not* sedative? This was a case of Rubeola Maligna, at the fourth day, with profound coma.—*E. M. Journal, February*, 1872.

Specific Medication.

(Synopsis of a Paper read before the Eclectic Medical Association of Ohio.)

GENTLEMEN:—At the last meeting of the State Society, I was requested to prepare a paper on Specific Medication, which should serve as a basis for a discussion of this new departure (as it has been called) in medicine.

I do not .propose, in doing this, to occupy much of your time in details, but rather to present the principles upon which specific or direct medication rests.

It will be well for us first, to think for a moment, (if it is possible for us to realize it), what an un-specific or indirect

medication is. It means that we never oppose remedies
directly to processes of disease, but on the contrary, influence diseased action in a roundabout, indirect, and uncertain
manner.

As examples—We violently excite the intestinal canal with
cathartics to arrest disease of the brain, the lungs, the kidneys,
or other distant parts. Or it is possible that we confine our
ministration first, to the gastric sac, then follow with potent
cathartics. In order, we excite the skin and the kidneys in
the same manner. This not sufficing, we counter-irritate
with rubefacients, blisters, etc., and so far as possible keep up
an influence counter to the disease by unpleasant, nauseating
and irritant medicines.

Whatever may be said in favor of such a practice, and how
fine-so-ever the theories with reference to it may be spun, it
is based upon the idea that two diseases can not exist in the
body at the same time, and if the medicines are sufficiently
potent, their action will surely be the strongest—and the disease will stop—leaving the patient to recover slowly from the
influence of the medicines.

Did you ever know the patient stop?—instead of the disease. I have, many a time, and have in this way, myself,
been a wonderful dispensation of Providence. In the olden
time men would not believe that the Doctors aided large
numbers of people out of the world. Oh no! The doctors,
God bless them, pulled the sick through; they would all
have died if it had not been for the Faculty.

It is wonderful how statistics take the conceit out of some
people and some things. When we find hundreds of cases of
severe disease tabulated—such as typhoid fever and pneumonia—with a mortality of but one to three per cent., with
only good nursing and food, no medicine; and active, potent
medication gives a mortality of five to fifty per cent.

Do Eclectic physicians kill people too? This brings the
matter home, and one doesn't like to confess his own sins, as
a rule. But in this matter I am like Artemus Ward in the
last war—I am willing to shed the blood of all my relations

—and I answer in the affirmative—they do kill—not so many as the old practice, it is true, but yet enough to cause us to look at home and rid ourselves of the evil.

Now I am glad to know that you, and Eclectics as a rule, have a very much better practice than theory. Whilst they occasionally wander off after these phantasms, it is the exception and not the rule.

As a body of physicians we recognize the fact that disease in all its forms is an impairment of life. And we recognize the necessity of conserving this life, and of employing such means as will increase it, and enable it to resist and throw off disease, and restore normal structure and function.

We recognize the importance of the functions of circulation, innervation, excretion, etc., and the necessity of obtaining as nearly a normal performance of them as possible. And all experience shows, that just in proportion as we get this normal performance, disease is arrested.

From its inception Eclecticism has been, to a very considerable extent, Specific Medication. The earliest writings point us to Dioscorea as a remedy for bilious colic, Hydrastis for enfeebled mucous membranes, Aralia and Apocynum for dropsy, Baptisia for putrid sore throat, and similar conditions of mucous membranes, Hamamelis for hemorrhoids, Macrotys for rheumatism, etc.

In our Materia Medicas, remedies were classed as Emetics, Cathartics, Diaphoretics, Tonics, Alteratives, etc., but in reading the description of medical properties, some special use or curative action would be pointed out, and for this it would be commonly used.

In all acute, and most chronic diseases, our examination of the patient and our therapeutics will take this order : 1. With reference to the condition of the stomach and intestinal canal —bringing them to as nearly a normal condition as possible, that remedies may be kindly received and appropriated, and that sufficient food may be taken and digested. 2. With reference to the circulation of the blood, and the temperature —obtaining a normal circulation as regards frequency and freedom, and a temperature as near 98° as possible. 3. With reference to the presence of a *zymotic* poison, or other cause of disease—which may be neutralized, antagonized or removed. 4. With reference to the condition of the nervous system—giving good innervation. 5. With reference to the processes of waste and excretion—that the worn out or enfeebled material may be broken down and speedily removed from the body. 6. With reference to blood-making and repair—that proper material be furnished for the building of tissue, and that the processes of nutrition are normally conducted.

We may illustrate this further by calling attention to the tongue as a means of diagnosing conditions of the stomach and intestinal canal, and of the blood.

You will bear in mind that diagnosis—or determining the real condition of disease is *the* most important part of Specific Medication. And that it is not that rough diagnosis which will enable us to guess off a *name* for the associated symptoms, at which name we will fire our Materia Medica promiscuously. Hence, when we question the tongue, it is not with reference to a remittent or typhoid fever, an inflammation of lungs, or rheumatism, but it is—I want you to tell me the condition of the stomach and intestinal canal, and especially the condition of the blood.

Now let us briefly see what it will tell us, with regard to the condition of the *primæ viæ:*

If the tongue is heavily coated at its base, with a yellowish-white fur, we know that there are morbid accumulations in the stomach; and we have to determine between the speedy removal by emesis, the slower removal by the Alkaline Sulphites, or the indirect removal by catharsis.

If the tongue is uniformly coated from base to tip with a yellowish fur, rather full, moist, we have the history of atony of the small intestine, and we give Podophyllin, Leptandrin, and this class of remedies with considerable certainty.

If the tongue is elongated and pointed, reddened at tip and *edges*, papillæ elongated and red, we have the evidence of irritation of the stomach with determination of blood. The therapeutics is plain : get rid of the irritation first, and be careful not to renew it by harsh medication.

Again, we have a tongue that might be designated as *slick*. It is variously colored, but it looks as if a fly should light on it he would slip up and break his neck. It is the evidence of a want of functional power, not only in the stomach and bowels, but of all parts supplied by sympathetic nerves. We treat such a case very carefully, avoid all irritants, and use means to restore innervation through the vegetative system of nerves.

The tongue tells us of acidity and alkalinity of the blood, and in language so plain that it can not be mistaken:

The *pallid* tongue, with white fur, is the index of acidity, and we employ an alkali—usually a salt of soda, with a certainty that the patient will be benefited. Indeed one who has never had his attention directed in this way, would be surprised at the improvement, in grave forms of disease, from one day's administration of simple Bicarbonate of Soda. 276

The *deep-red* tongue indicates alkalinity, and we prescribe an acid with a positive assurance that it will prove beneficial. Grave cases of typhoid fever and other zymotic diseases, presenting this symptom, have been treated with Acids alone, and with a success not obtained by other means. But it makes no difference what the disease is, whether a recent diarrhœa, or a grave typhoid dysentery, if there is the deep-red tongue, we give Muriatic Acid with the same assurance of success.

Impairment of the blood—sepsis—is indicated by *dirty coat-* ing, and by dark-colored fur—brownish to black. When we have either the one or the other we employ those remedies which antagonize the septic process.

The bitter tonics are indicated by fullness of tissue, with evident relaxation, impairment of circulation and muscular movement. The same condition will be an indication for

24

Iron. We give Tincture of Chloride of Iron if the tongue is red, Iron by Hydrogen if the tongue is pale.

The pale trembling tongue is a very good indication for the Hypophosphites.

The pale bluish tongue, expressionless, is the indication for the administration of Copper.

The dusky swollen tongue demands Baptisia.

You will notice that we have made this "unruly member" tell us a good deal, yet it might tell us more—it will tell us more when we thoroughly study it. My object is not to point out all that we might learn from it, but to show that it is possible to arrive at positive conclusions, from symptoms that are always definite in their meaning.

In making our diagnosis we question every function in the same way. We make the pulse tell us the condition of the circulation, and to some extent the nervous system that supplies it. We question the nervous system, the secretory organs—in fact every part.

One might suppose that diagnosis in this way would be a matter of great difficulty, as would the therapeutics based upon it, from the large number of remedies needed to meet these varying conditions of the several functions. But this is not so. On the contrary, the method is not only direct and certain, but it is easy.

We have but one life, though its manifestations are so varied. The control of this life is centered in a common nervous system—the ganglionic—and through this the various parts and functions are united. Disease is an aberration of this life—life in a wrong direction. Though it manifests itself in various ways, and though we study in detail as I have named, it is to grasp it at last as a unit, and oppose to it one or more remedies.

In some cases we have a first preparatory treatment, to fit the patient for the reception of remedies which directly oppose disease. As when we give an emetic to remove morbid accumulations, or means to relieve irritation of the stomach, or give an Acid or an Alkali, or use Veratrum and

Aconite to reduce frequency of pulse and temperature, to obtain the kindly action of Quinine in intermittent or remittent fever.

In other cases there are certain prominent symptoms indicating pathological conditions which may be taken as the key-notes of the treatment. As, when we have the full, open pulse, indicating Veratrum; the hypochondriac fullness, umbilical pains, and sallowness of skin, indicating Nux Vomica; the bright eye, contracted pupil and flushed face, calling for Gelseminum; or the dull eye, immobile pupil tendency to drowsiness, which calls for Belladonna.

In some cases the indication for a special remedy, like one of these, is so marked, that we give it alone, and it quickly cures most severe and obstinate diseases.

I would like to continue this subject further, for it is one in which I am greatly interested, and I know it is one in which you are interested, but the shortness of our session will not permit further remarks. But when we come together another year, with another year's experience, we may discuss it again.—*E. M. Journal, September*, 1871.

Elements of Uncertainty in Medicine.

The practice of medicine is proverbially uncertain, not so much possibly as regards the termination of disease, as regards the influence of medicine to palliate or arrest it. Instead of making this uncertainty a cardinal doctrine, a belief in which is absolutely essential to *regularity*, it seems to me it would be profitable to examine it carefully, and by analysis determine the "elements of uncertainty;" we might then hope to determine the "elements of certainty," and by a simple process of reasoning, avoid error and attain truth.

The most important factor in "medical uncertainty," is undoubtedly our present nosology. It is thought to be the chief end of medical study to attain such skill in diagnosis, that the diseases met with may be correctly classified, according to Good, Wood, Da Costa, or others. And having thus affixed a name by which they may be known, treat that name according to a Materia Medica which reads—"this remedy has been found useful in"—or "this remedy may be employed in," etc.

The element of uncertainty lies here, that a name employed to designate a disease, may cover the most diverse pathological states. The case of to-day, and the case of to-morrow, though justly called by the same name, may require a widely different treatment; the remedies employed successfully in one, would increase the disease in the other. Every one of our readers may draw the evidence of the truth of these propositions from his own practice.

The second "element of uncertainty" we find in the doctrine of idiosyncrasy, which is also a cardinal article of faith. We are gravely taught that in medicine one of nature's laws—that "like causes produce like effects," is inoperative; and, on the contrary, "that no man can possibly tell from the action of a medicine on one, what will be its influence upon another." The doctrine of idiosyncrasies is broad enough to cover all shortcomings and failures. And if true, then now and forever medicine will be a great uncertainty.

The third "element of uncertainty" lies in the application of the Latin motto, *post hoc ergo propter hoc*—that which follows a medicine must be due to its influence. If a man recovers from sickness after taking Podophyllin or Quinine, it is due to these agents, and he probably would not have gotten well without them. But there is this singular fact here: whilst physicians are willing to credit their remedies with all relief from suffering, improvement and restoration to health, they are not willing to reverse it, and concede increase of suffering, prolongation of disease and death to the remedies, though the sequence is quite as natural in the one case as the other.

It does seem strange that physicians should have so thoroughly believed that medicine *saved* the lives of the sick, that without it the majority, or all, would have died. Strange that they never should have observed, until within the past score of years, that abundant provision might have been made by the Creator for the removal of disease, and that it was possible that medicine might be adding to the death-rate, rather than lessening it. Even now when all this is proven beyond cavil, by some of the best observers, we find the majority won't believe it; even if they concede it in theory, they deny it in practice.

The fourth element of uncertainty lies in the endeavor to get direct results from indirect agencies. You want to influence the circulation and the temperature, and you give remedies which produce emesis or catharsis. You want to elect Greeley, and you whip your neighbor because he "rah's" for Grant.

The fifth element of uncertainty is the administration of remedies in poisonous instead of medicinal doses. It is true that the poisonous action may be known with some certainty, but its influence upon disease is very uncertain.

The poisonous action sets up a new process of disease in so far as it changes structure and function, and it may be curative according to the law of substitution. A medicinal action we understand to be one that restores function, and thus removes disease.

Give your remedy in medicinal doses, and then you may expect direct and positive results in the relief of disease.

These are the principal elements of uncertainty in regular medicine and in our school. To these we might add a number of minor ones, among which is a belief in "special providences," inscrutable or otherwise. Indeed any one who is inclined to shift his responsibility upon his Creator, and to believe that the laws of nature can be suspended from any *providence*, has all the elements of uncertainty with him.

The principal element of uncertainty in Homœopathic medicine is the making of *pain* a principal symptom, and the treatment of symptoms in place of pathological conditions. The cheerful trust in Nature of the high dilutionist is laudable, though we can't say so much for their claim to all the glory of relief and recovery.

This is but a rough sketch of the subject, which we present as good material for thought. We purpose using it as a text in the future, and elaborating some of the points. In our next article, we will consider the "elements of certainty" in medicine, in the same order.—*E. M. Journal, July,* 1872.

Elements of Certainty in Medicine.

In our last article we briefly discussed the "elements of uncertainty in medicine," and we now propose to look at the other side—how may we attain certainty in medicine. We all agree that the practice of medicine in the past has been notoriously uncertain, and that there is yet great room for improvement.

The first, and most important element of "uncertainty" is found in our present nosology, and the constant tendency to prescribe for names of disease. The first "element of certainty" will be, therefore, an entire avoidance of this error, diagnosing pathological conditions and prescribing for these.

We have heretofore seen that disease, as we meet it in the individual, consists of a series of functional lesions—all disease is an impairment of function. Certain prominent lesions or symptoms give a name to the disease, according to the present nosology, but the name does not, and can not convey to the mind the character of the lesions or the treatment required to remove them. If I say my patient has "pneumonia" (taking one of the simplest diseases), I give you no information which would guide you to a correct treatment, and if you prescribe it must be upon the idea that all inflammations of the lung are alike, unless you follow the expectant plan, and use the "mush poultice," with rest and good nursing.

In one case the prominent lesion would be of the circulation and temperature; and we would stop the inflammation by the third day with the use of Veratrum and the bath, alone. In another case with small pulse, and tendency to congestion, we would relieve our patient speedily with the use of Aconite and Belladonna, and the local application of

Compound Powder of Lobelia to the chest. In a third class of cases, with especial impairment and feebleness of mucous structure, Ipecac would be a prominent remedy. In a fourth class of cases, with special impairment of skin and dryness of mucous membranes, we would use Asclepias. In a fifth, if we had the broad *pallid* tongue, we might treat the case with Bicarbonate of Soda alone. In a sixth, of typhoid character, we would obtain especial benefit from Sulphurous Acid, Muriatic Acid, Sulphite of Soda, or Baptisia. In a seventh class of cases, with hypochondriac fullness, umbilical pain, sallowness and puffiness of skin, yellowness about the mouth, and the coloring matter of bile in urine, I will cure every case with the single remedy, Nux Vomica. Eighth, all our readers know that there is a class of cases in which Quinine is eminently curative, and will alone speedily arrest the disease.

Is it not most absurd, therefore, to talk about a stereotyped treatment of pneumonia? We have named eight classes of cases, and in the entire lot have wanted no remedy for the lungs. It really makes no difference whether it is an inflammation of the lungs or the nates, only in so much as a man breathes with the one and sits on the other.

Specific diagnosis is therefore the first element of certainty in medicine. We want to know the character of the lesion of the circulation, the temperature, the functions of digestion, nutrition, secretion and excretion. innervation, etc., and knowing these, and how remedies influence these functions, we prescribe with a reasonable degree of certainty.

The second element of certainty is a firm reliance on nature's law—"that like causes produce like effects." We are not looking for "idiosyncrasies" to excuse our ignorance, or "special or inscrutable providences" to cover our defects and shortcomings. We want to study those symptoms and signs that determine exact conditions of disease, and then knowing the action of remedies we may always give them with certainty.

The third element of uncertainty we found to be the taking

of every good result that followed the administration of a remedy, as being due to its action. This must be carefully avoided. We study the direct or specific action of remedies by using them singly, and observing the consequences in numerous cases; it is confessedly a work of time, and a work of difficulty, but it can be done.

The fourth element of certainty is found in giving remedies for their direct effects, and not as they produce counter-irritation or some other disease. If the circulation is wrong, we give a remedy that acts directly upon the circulatory system, and in such way that the wrong may be righted. If there is a lesion of the blood, we give a remedy that reaches the blood and antagonizes the lesion. If the skin, kidneys or bowels fail to do their work of excretion, we reach them by remedies that exert their influence directly, and so of the entire Materia Medica.

The fifth element of certainty consists in the use of remedies in medicinal doses and for their direct curative influence. No man can tell what influence an active cathartic will have upon a frequent circulation, any more than he can tell what the influence of a blister will be in pneumonia. The course of a medicinal disease is notoriously uncertain, as is exampled by the use of mercurials.

A sixth element of certainty, and a very important one is—that we have reliable medicines. If we are to take our remedies "hit or miss" from the drug trade, our practice will be "hit or miss." The drugs of the market are notoriously uncertain. We want our indigenous remedies gathered at the proper season, and prepared for use from the fresh or recent articles. The best form is a fluid preparation, of the strength of eight ounces Troy to the pint of product. This can be kept from season to season, is uniform in strength, easily dispensed, pleasant on account of smallness of dose, and reliable in its action. Without uniformly good preparations, the practice of medicine must be uncertain, and there will be a constant tendency to gross medication and drugging.—*E. M. Journal, August,* 1872.

The Doctrine of Substitution.

In the olden time the doctrine of substitution was a prominent feature with some Eclectics. They could see no need of any change in the commonly received doctrine of the Old School, and they were firm believers in phlogosis and antiphlogistics. Blood-letting, Mercury and Antimony, etc., were an offence to them—not because of their general depressant influence, but because they were thought to be unmanageable, or exerted some special or permanent pernicious influence.

When the writer attended his lectures, this doctrine of substitution was prominently brought forward, and lecturers would labor to show that we had substitutes for the old means, quite as effectual at the time, but transient in action.

There were a number of substitutes for bloodletting. Prof. Buchanan spent much time in showing how *hemastasis* could be employed, even to the extent of syncope in active inflammation, and when we had obtained the desired influence, the blood could be gradually let back from the corded limbs into the general circulation, and thus whilst we had obtained the antiphlogistic influence of bloodletting in the relief of inflammation, we had saved the vital fluid. "The boy had eaten his cake and saved it."

Profs. Jones and Morrow believed that all the good effects of bloodletting could be obtained by vigorous cathartics; that in this free catharsis the bloodvessels could be depleted almost as quickly, and to a far greater extent, whilst the vital portions of the blood were saved, and the serum would be quickly renewed.

Prof. Cleveland and some others thought that this influence could be obtained by the kidneys as well as the bowels, and that the two at least were equal to bloodletting. Whilst in addition, you would be promoting the removal of large quantities of effete material.

Mercury, in the form of Blue-pill, Calomel, etc., was the

25

Samson of regular practice, acting on the liver and thus removing disease. We must have a substitute for this Samson, for we too must "touch the liver" of our patients. And it was claimed that in Podophyllum and Podophyllin we had a greater than Samson, or if we wanted the certain but mild action on the liver—like blue-pill—we would use Leptandra or Leptandrin. But we must "tap the liver," and thus we could do it safely.

But these would not "touch the gums," and as our opponents regarded "touching the gums" as essential to the successful treatment of some diseases, we must find a substitute for Mercury in this direction, and touch the gums too. For this purpose Iris was recommended, or equal parts of Iridin, Podophyllin and Xanthoxylum, given in grain doses every hour or two. And we are told "that salivation from vegetable agents may be known from that by Mercury, by the absence of mercurial fetor, and no sponginess of the gums or loosening of the teeth." And that when Eclectics, from having produced such salivation, are unjustly accused of using Mercury, they may excuse themselves by calling attention to the above differences.

The necessity of vigorous counter-irritation by gut and skin was recognized, and many similar means were employed to obtain it. "Profound impression," by active cathartics, was required in the treatment of many diseases, and for this purpose we would take Gamboge, Scammony, Colocynth, etc., and make the combination Eclectic by adding Podophyllum or other indigenous remedy. We *must* use the blister, and Cantharides being the only certain agent, at least the only one that could be handled with safety, we take it. But as it would not do to go too far in this direction, we substituted for the Tartar Emetic ointment, a vegetable irritating plaster.

Nauseant expectorants must be used in diseases of the respiratory organs, and we substituted for Tartar Emetic, Lobelia and Sanguinaria, but we still retained Ipecac. Stimulant expectorants must be used, and we kept Squills, Senega, Tolu, etc., because we had none better, and thus the doctrine of substitution ramified in every direction, and in some cases it would be so slight that there would be no real difference.

Was this Eclecticism? Do you think it possible that a School of Medicine, increasing for thirty years, could be founded on so small a basis? These were errors that grew out of a want of a well defined statement of principles, and especially a want of knowledge on the part of some teachers.

There was a profound conviction that the old depressant practice was wholly wrong, and that in its stead treatment should be restorative. So that really whilst substitution was thus freely talked of, entirely different means were employed. Just in proportion as the practitioner departed from the old ideas and methods, and employed restorative means, just in that proportion he was successful.

But it was not only the rejection of the antiphlogistic plan, and the recognition of Nature in the cure of disease, that gave impetus to the Eclectic movement. But beyond this, and fully as important was the introduction of new remedies, for their direct action in opposing and removing disease. Take the Medical Reformer in its five volumes, and all our earlier medical publications, and you will find a large list of remedies that had been carefully studied, and the use of which gave great success in practice. These earlier Eclectics taught Specific Medication as certainly as has Dr. Scudder, though they did not use the name. And what is more, they obtained just the same influences from many of them that he has, and they describe this action in just the same way.

It need hardly be added, that those earlier publications of our School, have been a mine of information which the writer has worked advantageously for the past dozen years.

This doctrine of substitution has been the bane of our School, constantly drawing us backwards. We want none of it. We do not believe the old doctrines of disease, we want no antiphlogistic or depressant treatment in any case. Eclectic medicine looks to the conservation of vital power, is restorative, and so far as possible advocates specific medicines for specific pathological conditions.—*E. M. J., June,* 1871.

Poison vs. Medicine.

As we have stated, "almost all drugs have two actions— a poisonous and a medicinal. We want to avoid the one and obtain the other." How shall we study the Materia Medica to obtain this desirable end?

At first thought it would seem that the difference between the poisonous and medicinal action was wholly one of dose. If I administer two grains of Strychnia I give a poison, if the one-thirtieth of a grain it favors life; if I give five grains of Morphia the patient dies, if but one-third of a grain he has refreshing sleep. You can kill a man with large doses of Podophyllin, Lobelia, Jalap, and a hundred agents of like character, when small doses would not kill, and might be medicinal.

But this is only partly true. The dose may be large enough to be poisonous, and then the size of the dose will be the only element of danger, but there is another consideration of more importance.

Those agencies that we call remedies exert an action upon the body, and change one or more of its functional activities. If we give a drug to a healthy person, it produces disease, and it is because it thus acts upon the body that it becomes a remedy—an agent that had no such action would be useless. To make this agent a remedy, however, it is essential that there should be a functional wrong of the part upon which this agent acts, and that its action opposes the wrong of disease, and favors the return to health.

If now we mistake, and give a medicine to influence a functional wrong that does not exist, then we are poisoning our patient—it may be slowly, but the influence is nevertheless poisonous.

To illustrate, we find a condition of the system in some malarious diseases in which Quinine is tolerated in large doses, and is curative. We give a dose of twenty grains in congestive remittent with the happiest results, because the remedy is antagonized by the disease; but under different circumstances the patient would suffer seriously.

We find cases in which patients can take large doses of the Bromides with safety and benefit for a long time, but in others the remedies are poisonous in moderate doses. I have seen serious results from the use of Iodide of Potassium for a long time, as I have from other remedies given by rote.

I have been censured for giving Copper as a remedy, because it was a poison. And yet we find pickles *greened* with Copper as an article of food on many tables for years. My use of Copper has been attended with the happiest results, and I use it with quite as clear a conscience as I use Iron, but I only use it when Copper is wanted.

I have been censured for the use of Bismuth, because it is not a constituent of the body, and yet I have never seen the harm following this agent, that I have from Podophyllin.

It has been clearly demonstrated within the past two years, that Phosphorus and Arsenic are very closely related chemically and medicinally. That Phosphorus exerts a very similar influence upon the skin, and may be used in place of Arsenic in skin diseases. Yet Phosphorus as Phosphorus is by far the most difficult to use, the most unmanageable, and the most likely to poison the patient, yet none of these rabid Eclectics object to the use of Phosphorus?

Why do I object to the use of Mercury? Because its influence is to impair the vitality of the body   It is destructive in its nature—and I want no remedies of this character. I object to the use of Antimony upon the same grounds, to the use of the lancet, the blister, harsh purgation, the entire class of antiphlogistics, from what ever source obtained. I base my objections upon principle, and not because there is a prejudice against these things. If I believed in the necessity of antiphlogistics, as some do, I should employ bloodletting and Mercury as the principal means, because they are the typical antiphlogistics, and will destroy life faster than any thing else.—*E. M. Journal, August*, 1872.

Treatment of Disease with a Single Remedy.

The perfection of specific medicine is found in those cases, in which the entire series of functional lesions is removed by *one* drug. Possibly medicine will never attain such perfection; it is possible we have quite as much knowledge now as we ever will have, but as we have some marked examples of this, it is reasonable to conclude that time will develop more.

In studying the specific action of Tinctura Ferri Chloridi we found some singular but well attested facts. We found that this remedy was specific in a majority of cases of erysipelas, and that in many of these its action could not be accounted for by the older therapeutic doctrines.

Here is a disease presenting all the functional lesions of the severest zymotic fever. A hot, dry skin, temperature of 106°, pulse 120 per minute, small and hard, mouth dry and parched, tongue brown, sordes on teeth, delirium, and an unpleasant local inflammation constantly spreading. We commence the administration of Tincture of Muriate of Iron in doses of ten drops. Before the second dose the effect is noticed, and within twenty-four hours, the pulse has fallen and become more natural, the temperature is reduced, the skin is soft and moist, the delirium has passed away, the patient has slept and is conscious, the mouth is moist, tongue cleaning, and the local inflammatory process arrested. In a few days the patient is convalescent, and yet but a single remedy has been given. It has been sedative, diaphoretic, diuretic, a nervine and an antizymotic, and a more efficient one than any that could be selected from the Materia Medica.

Every one of our readers knows these facts with regard to Iron, in the treatment of some cases of this disease. Is Iron in erysipelas an anomaly in therapeutics, the one exception to all general rules?

Let us take Quinine as another example, and I will try to give a case that the majority of my readers have seen—one of malarial pneumonia. The patient was attacked with a severe chill, followed by fever, increasing from day to day. There was at first an irritative cough, followed by soreness of chest, difficult breathing, rusty sputa, and the usual physical signs. Severe from the commencement, it was only aggravated by the expectorants *ad nauseam*, the cathartics, blister, and associate means. Now the ninth day of the disease there is purulent expectoration, great prostration, and the evidences of early dissolution. Doctors are changed, and the new one recognizes it as a case for Quinia. There is relief from the first dose, and a rapid amendment and convalescence in a few days.

I name this case, because it is one I have seen within the last few weeks, but the reader can recall many cases of a similar kind. Here Quinine has been everything that is good, sedative, diaphoretic, diuretic, stimulant, tonic, a remedy for the lungs, the *one* thing necessary.

I have just completed the treatment of one of the severest cases of cardítis, associated with inflammation of the posterior portion of the lung, that I have ever met with, in which the action of Quinine at a certain stage was quite as marked. The patient had been under *regular* treatment, with consult-ations for eight days, when he came into my hands. There was disturbance of the bowels, demanding special treatment, an unpleasant circulation, effusion into the pericardium, and delirium, all of which seemed to demand something. By the end of the week, I saw the place for Quinine, and with four doses of a grain each, daily, and small doses of Cactus, all the symptoms rapidly faded away. It relieved the delirium, gave sleep, quieted the cough, brought the pulse down and gave it regularity, established secretion, and did all that was necessary. And I may state this important fact, the patient was *not* convalescing when it was commenced, but had had a severe relapse.

Now I would hardly undertake to point out the symptoms that caused me to give the Quinine in this case. There was no malarial poison, nothing seemingly for it to antidote, but there was an impairment of the nervous system for which ;

was *the* remedy. I admit that I should be able to point out the symptoms so that another could recognize the case, and tell *why* I give Quinine in certain cases, as in the one above, but I can't as yet.

We will sometimes find quite as marked examples in the administration of Nux Vomica. I recall a case in the past year of severe fever at the fifth day, not controlled in the least by the sedatives and associate means. A peculiar yellowness about mouth, umbilical pains, with increasing nausea, caused me to give Nux Vomica. The prescription was: ℞ Tinct. Nux Vomica, gtts. v.; Water, ℥iv.; a teaspoonful every hour. The next morning there was a decided amelioration in all the symptoms, and by the seventh day the patient was convalescent. So I have treated inflammation of the lungs, fever, dysentery, colic, diarrhœa, and many other named diseases, with Nux alone, the symptoms pointing to it distinctly, and with the most satisfactory results.

Doubtless, most of our readers have noticed a peculiarity of pulse, to which Aconite is *the* remedy. And with Aconite alone have been able to treat the entire disease with more than ordinary success. Given the small pulse, with moderate hardness, and a singular vibration like a violin string under the finger, and we have as near as I can give it the indication. To be plain, I say give Aconite always when the pulse is *small* and frequent, but sometimes it is only one of a number of remedies necessary, but in some it is *all*. Now let us learn to know those cases in which it is *all*, and then we will obtain the same results as we see from Quinine when it is specific.

There is a condition of disease to which Baptisia is specific in the same way. My first experience with this was in the Winter of 1859, in an endemic of cynanche maligna. In some of these cases the symptoms were as grave as in typhoid fever, and the ordinary treatment was not a success. Yet Baptisia controlled the frequency of pulse, lessened the temperature, established secretion, restored digestion, antidoted the rapid sepsis, and controlled the local disease. I have given it in three cases of typhoid fever with like results. There were

characteristic symptoms indicating the use of the remedy,
and when given it checked irritation of the bowels, lessened
the fever, stopped the progress of sepis—indeed, did all for
the patients that the most sanguine could have asked. I
have used it in one case of dysentery (alone) with like results.
Some of our Homœopathic friends up North give their testimony in its favor, giving a large number of cases like the
above, so that it has not been a single experience. And I find
on reading back, that Eclectics had similar results twenty-
five years since.

We can reach but one conclusion from this, and that is,
that there is a condition of disease to which Baptisia is specific, and when this condition is the basis of the series of
morbid processes that make the disease before us, it may be
the *one* remedy for the totality of disease.

I have been guided by two symptoms, the peculiar fullness
and purplish discoloration of fauces and pharynx, and the
papescent, frothy, dark-colored feces. That there are others,
I doubt not, and probably some more positive, but these
would cause me to give Baptisia in any case.

I have seen the gravest forms of disease rapidly fade away,
upon the administration of Bi-carbonate of Soda when the
common means had failed. There was a special indication
for it; any one might see it, if he knew how and where to
look. And now simple Soda becomes sedative where sedatives had failed, gives sleep where Opium had failed, estab-
lishes secretion, antidotes the blood-poison, or is actually
antiperiodic where Quinine has proven a failure. In evidence
I may cite Prof. King, who gave me my first instruction in
this, and might add hundreds of others.

If we wanted evidence badly, I might bring forward
Chambers, Anstie, Bennett, Wunderlich, and others, to prove
that very similar results have been obtained from the use of
Muriatic Acid. With it alone, hundreds, yes, thousands of
cases of typhoid and typhus fever have been treated, with a
mortality ranging from less than one per cent. to never more
than three. There was something special in these diseases

that the Acid met, and it was the *one* thing necessary, *everything* necessary. We have learned to determine this condition and we use Acids in a rational way.

I might give other examples, but these will suffice to awaken attention, and all that the subject wants is thought and investigation. There is here a broad field for study, and one that should well repay research. That medicine will ever reach such perfection, that we will be able to select *one* remedy for the totality of disease in all cases, I do not believe, but that it may be done in a considerable number, I am quite certain.—*E. M. Journal, June,* 1872.

Pleasant Medicines.

The great desideratum in the practice of medicine is pleasant remedies. In the olden times, and with many now, medicine adds to the sufferings of the sick, and they dread more the unpleasantness of the doctor's prescriptions than they do the disease.

In looking over our Materia Medicas and Dispensatories, it would seem that our object has been to make the concoctions as nauseous as possible. In extemporaneous prescriptions it is the same; the combination of remedies, and the vehicle, combine to make the mixture unpleasant.

It has been thought that sugar or syrup would cover up the unpleasantness of medicine, and hence it is most commonly used. The fact is, however, that with the majority of the sick the sweet is unpleasant, and nothing could be more objectionable than a nauseous sweet. The doctor don't take his own medicines, and hence he does not know how objectionable they are, and he continues giving these unpleasant mixtures year after year, to the detriment of his patient, and his own pocket.

Let us first get rid of the idea that medicines should be and can be *disguised*. It never had one atom of truth in it, and a very little experimentation will determine its falsity. Take anything that is unpleasant, and the more you disguise it the worse it is. Some medicines are very objectionable in their taste, but they are less disgusting to the patient alone, than when mixed with syrup or other vehicle.

The *best* form of vegetable remedies is a simple tincture by percolation: the best form for all remedies, if possible, is the fluid form. It is not only the best as regards the medicinal action of the remedy, but is also the pleasantest as well.

The *best* vehicle for the administration of a remedy, is water, and it also is the pleasantest. But few remedies are intended to exert a local influence upon the mucous coat of the stomach. All others must first gain entrance to the circulation, before their curative action can be obtained. To get into the blood by osmose, it is necessary that the agent be in solution, and of less specific gravity than the blood. If you do not have your remedy in solution before its administration, its getting into the circulation will depend upon the stomach supplying the necessary amount of fluid and effecting the solution.

To the sick, there are but few of our remedies objectionable, if they are properly prepared with alcohol and given with water. The dose of properly prepared remedies is quite small, so that, added to fresh water in such proportion that the dose will be a teaspoonful, it is much diluted. Even if the taste is objectionable, there is evidence of cleanliness, and nothing to disgust.

For years, I have made my prescriptions in one way—to a glass of fresh water adding the necessary amount of tincture or fluid medicine to make the dose a teaspoonful. In acute diseases the dose should be frequently repeated, hence it is necessarily small. Of a strong tincture of Aconite or Veratrum. gtts. v. to gtts. xx. to ℥iv.; of Gelseminum, ℨj. to ℥iv.; of Macrotys, Asclepias, Lobelia, etc., ℨj. to ℥iv. As a rule, these doses exert a more marked curative effect than the larger ones commonly given.

But it is in the treatment of children that unpleasant medicine is most objectionable. It is not pleasant to see the little ones start with distrust when the doctor makes his appearance, nor to be obliged to force medicines upon a child. We get along much better if we have the confidence of the children, and it is certainly much pleasanter.

I always prepare the medicines before my little patients. They see the water is fresh, their medicine looks clean and nice, whilst its quantity is small, and the mixture does not look objectionable. They taste it when asked, taking the first dose from the doctor, and give their opinion decidedly that it is good, (or at least not bad), and after this they take it kindly as the hour comes around.—*E. M. Journal, January*, 1871.

Conservation of Life.

It is fortunate for mankind that we have *life* enough to resist processes of disease, and the medicaments of the doctor. This power of resistance, and vital tenacity, is really one of the most wonderful facts of our existence, and should be an admirable argument in the hand of the theologian to prove the fore-knowledge of the Creator. It is the salvation of physic—for if it were not for this strong tenacity, doctors would soon bury all their patrons, and have to seek other means of livelihood.

In some seasons, we have this subject forced upon our attention in a way that we can not avoid it, and we are obliged to learn a lesson whether we will or no. As an example, some physicians have learned this season, for the first time, that Quinine will not cure all cases of ague, and that it will act as a poison, leaving effects that are never recovered from.

So many learn the necessity of conserving the life, carefully guarding the feeble flame, and strengtening it, from some endemic or epidemic disease of an asthenic character which they see for the first time. The experience comes to some with dysentery, in others with inflammation of the lungs, typhoid fever, or even in the ordinary " bilious " fevers of our country. One lesson is sufficient for many, but the most of us require more ; but when we have these experiences, and the fact is *forced* on our attention, our practice undergoes a change, and we become very conservative.

This experience has come to a great many this year, and we hear of it constantly in letters coming to our office. To many it has come through the typho-malarial fever so prevalent this fall, in which even the simplest depressants—purgatives for instance—have been sufficient to produce death.

I give an instance from my own practice as an example—the only fatal case out of seventeen cases of this severe fever:

Was called to see patient who had been sick with this fever for fifteen days, "given up" by the attending physician, and was not expected to live out the twenty-four hours. Careful attention, conserving life, was followed by recovery, though it required five more weeks. In the second week of my attendance, two more children took the disease, and though I did my best, the fever would run its course, and presently I was satisfied with holding my own—conserving life, in their cases. Both were convalescent the fourth week. But in the meanwhile a fourth child took the fever, not worse than the others, seemingly stouter, and having more vital tenacity. The sick in that house were getting too thick, and I concluded that in at least one of the cases I ought to stop the disease with medicine. The tongue was fearfully *dirty*, abdomen tumid, and I concluded to cleanse the *primæ viæ* with a cathartic—the child was dead in three days. Instead of cleansing the "way of life," I wiped it out. There was no other reason why the boy should not have lived as did his brothers and sister, and he would have lived, in all probability, if he had had the same treatment.

It is not pleasant to sit in judgment on oneself, but I have found it profitable. I know there is no mean between good and harm in medicine as we use it; it will do one or the other—if it does not oppose disease, it opposes life. I know this talk about idiosyncrasy is all bosh, and when a medicine does harm, I am to blame, not the patient; and I try to learn a lesson from it, and not to fall into the same error again.—*E. M. Journal, December*, 1871.

On the Use of Restoratives.

In order that the body may properly perform its functions, it is necessary that there shall be normal nutrition of tissue. Life grows out of the continued change of matter, and it is active and healthy in proportion to the decomposition and recomposition of tissue.

The food taken each twenty-four hours represents the force required and used in its organization, and used in the human body this force is set free as needed, and is living force. Just as in the wood burned under the steam-boiler, there is locked up the force required for its organization, derived from the sun, and which in the process of burning is set free, and manifests itself to us in the steam engine as power.

If from any cause we have an impairment of nutrition, we must have an impairment of life in the same proportion, manifesting itself in simple deficiency of function, or in its perversion.

Certainly in any such case the restoration of normal nutrition is one of the most important indications of treatment. And in the majority, we will find that as we approximate normal nutrition, we return to the condition of health.

If we have an impairment of nutrition, what shall we do? You answer—give *bitter tonics and iron.* But experience proves that this is not always good practice, and if we would think for a moment we would see that it is very unphilosophical. Bitter tonics are mostly gastric stimulants, increasing the appetite and to a limited extent gastric digestion. Iron is required for the building of red-globules. This it will be noticed is but a small part of what we have to take into consideration.

In studying nutrition and its derangements, we have to consider: 1st. The food, that it is good, properly proportioned between the histogenetic and calorifacient, and that it contains all the elements of the tissues in proper proportion and in such form that it can be appropriated. 2d. That the action of digestion—buccal, stomachic and intestinal—shall be properly performed. 3d. That the blood is free from effete material, in regular circulation, and the associate blood-making organs are working well. 4th. The material being properly prepared, and taken to the part, that the part itself is in condition to appropriate it. (*a.*) That the old tissues are removed. (*b.*) That the formative force is sufficient for cell reproduction.

We see that the lesion of nutrition may be dependent upon a wrong in the food; upon a lesion of digestion—either buccal, gastric, or intestinal; upon effete material in the blood; upon an impairment of the circulation; upon a deficiency of formative force in the cells of the part; or upon a defect of waste, the old tissues not being broken down and carried away.

It may be rectified by selecting proper food, by such elemental substances as are necessary to nutrition, or by getting good mastication and insalivation, or by those agents which facilitate gastric digestion, or by those which facilitate intestinal digestion, or by those which remove effete material from the blood, or by those which favor an equal and uniform circulation of the blood, or by those which stimulate the formative act in the tissues, or by those which aid the process of retrograde metamorphosis—removing the old tissues.—*E. M. Journal, April*, 1871.

Pain and its Treatment.

What is health? That condition of body in which all functions are a source of pleasure. What must then be the condition when the performance of function, or simple existence, is unpleasant? Disease. We say a person *suffers* from disease, and the language of the people correctly expresses the fact—disease is a condition of suffering, or suffering is a condition of disease. If people did not *suffer* in disease, they would think very much less of it than they do, and might bear the confinement with considerable equanimity.

We ask the question, again—What influence has the ordi-

nary practice of medicine upon the unpleasantness of disease
that we call suffering? Let us think for a moment, before
answering this question, and see if we can call up a past experience in our own bodies to aid in solving the question.
How is it with Castor Oil, Jalap and Senna, Podophyllin, a
pint of Polygonum Punctatum or Eupatorium, a nauseant of
Lobelia, Ipecac, Sanguinaria, *et id omne genus?* In the
ordinary use of medicines do we increase the unpleasantness
of disease?

In the olden time this was thought necessary to *save* life,
but we now know that this was a professsonal fiction, and that
instead of *saving* life, mortality was increased by this use of
medicines. Unpleasantness and suffering are evidences of
disease—impairment of life—increase these by medicines,
and you increase the sum of disease, and still further impair
life.

We conclude from this that a *correct* practice of medicine
should be pleasant in itself, and that it should look to removing unpleasantness and suffering, for these are evidences of
disease.

Admitting that it is still necessary to produce a temporary
increase of suffering, to remove the cause of a more prolonged
suffering, as when we give an emetic, or a cathartic of Podophyllin, we want to restrict these necessities as much as possible, and finally get rid of them if we can.

But there are times when the suffering in disease becomes
unbearable, the patient must have rest and relief from pain,
and for this purpose we are presented with certain drugs
which obtund sensibility—called narcotics. Really, these
consist of Opium and its salts, and the new agent, Hydro-
chloral. So great is the seeming necessity for these, that the
imports of the first amount to some millions of dollars yearly,
and the second is weighed by *tons.* They are in such common
use, and regarded as so indispensable, that we find them on
every physician's shelves, and in every pocket case and pill-
bags, and prescribed on every page of a druggist's prescrip-
tion-book.

To these remedies, and to this common use I object, and I propose to give these objections "form and comeliness," and if possible present a better way.

I object to the ordinary use of narcotics, because they are prescribed for symptoms and not for conditions of disease. It is well known by all who have studied modern. pathology, that pain and sleeplessness may be due to two distinct and opposite conditions of the brain. In the one case the condition is *active*—irritation and determination of blood. In the other, the condition is one of *atony*—the circulation and nutrition being enfeebled. Clearly these two conditions require different treatment—for which will you prescribe Opium? and what will you do for the other?

You find your patient alike sleepless in these two opposite conditions. In one the skin is dry and harsh, temperature high, pulse frequent and hard, secretions arrested. In the other the pulse is small and feeble, the face pallid, and the extremities cold. In which of these cases will you give Opium? and what will you do for the other?

You find severe pain in a part, the patient wants relief, must have rest; did it ever suggest itself to you that it was worth while to take into consideration the condition of the part—whether it was one of *activity or atony*, or the general conditions as named above? In the ordinary use of narcotics these things are not considered, and hence the common use of these drugs is the worst form of empiricism.

I have nothing to say about the uncertainty of their action, and the ill effects so frequently following their use. Every reader has had these experiences, and I have no doubt, would be only too glad to know how to get along without them, or learn to use them with greater certainty.

I recognize the fact that there are two factors in this problem of unpleasantness—pain, sleeplessness. The one is the general condition of the body, embracing every function; the other is the condition of the brain and its sensitive nerves. And I formulize it in this way. As is the departure from the normal standard of health in function and condition, so will

26

be the unpleasantness, pain, sleeplessness. Conversely, when we have either of these, we may expect relief just in proportion as we restore the body to its normal condition, and the brain to its normal condition.

Thus, when my patient is suffering, or sleepless, I determine as near as may be, what derangement of function is the cause, and instead of prescribing narcotics, I adopt those means that restore the diseased function.

If the condition is one of irritation and determination of blood to the brain, relief and sleep come from the use of the sedatives and Gelseminum. If the condition is one of atony, it comes from the use of stimulants, tonics, and food.

Prescribing for the *basic* element of disease, is a very certain way of relieving pain and giving sleep. You will get those results from the simple administration of Bicarbonate of Soda, Muriatic Acid, Sulphuric Acid, Baptisia, Phytolacca, when these are specially indicated, as well as from the use of remedies that more especially influence the nervous system.

Hoping that I have at least placed this subject in such light that our readers can think of it, and solve the problem for themselves, we will leave it for this time. I may remark, in conclusion, that I have not given a narcotic in eighteen months, and have not used the equivalent of a drachm of Morphia in five years.—*E. M. Journal, April,* 1872.

Diagnosis and Treatment of Obscure Cases.

We all have our troublesome cases, in which the symptoms are not pronounced, and the diagnosis is obscure, and the treatment being guess-work, proves a failure. The best men may make mistakes in diagnosis, but it should be of rare occurrence, and never one that will lead to the improper administration of medicine.

Let us take a single condition of the intestinal canal as an example. We are sent for to see a patient, and find him confined to room or bed, and complaining of inaction of the bowels. Question him as you will, the end is the same—constipation—and he feels certain if his bowels are moved, all will be well. Will we give him a physic? And continue to repeat it, increasing its strength?

Not by any means. We see in constipation but a symptom, and not one especially indicating the character of the disease. It might be the disease called "bilious colic." I have seen it with a *very* moderate amount of pain; and though Compound Powder of Jalap, in broken doses, would prove curative, Podophyllin and the harsher cathartics would kill. It might be acute enteritis, and then the dry skin, small, hard pulse, white narrow tongue, tenderness on deep pressure, would determine the character of the disease; and we would *not* give a cathartic under any circumstances. Again it might be hernia—some of the obscurer forms, or ileus—invagination, in either case, a cathartic would be the worst medicine we could give.

In the above cases the constipation seems to be the direct symptom, if it is not the disease itself. So in many other cases, the symptoms that seem to point out the disease, are quite as likely to lead to wrong as right treatment.

Supposing we take pain in the bowels—colic, as another example. It won't do, to depend upon the character of the pain always, to tell us the lesion or the proper remedy—and it don't do to call it colic, and prescribe at random. As an example, I was called to see a case that had been under the care of a Homœopath, who prescribed for the character of the pain; but the woman had suffered intensely for hours, and was exhausted by the severity of the pain. The inhalation of Chloroform for ten minutes gave entire relief, and there was no return of pain—there was intestinal spasm. Another: I had prescribed for a case of abdominal pain, in the early part of my practice, the usual routine of aromatics, stimulants, chloroform by mouth, winding up with Compound Powder of Jalap, until the stomach refused to tolerate any more medicine—and all without relief. A Homœopathic practitioner was called, and prescribing Nux Vomica alone, had the patient comfortable in three or four hours. I might

have done it, as well as he, if I had known then what I know
now.   The peculiar yellowness around mouth, sense of fullness and oppression in right hypochondrium, and pain pointing at umbilicus, told the story clearly.   I recollect a case of
green apples in my boyhood, and the drenching with Com-
position and diluted No. 6, as prescribed by a disciple of
Samuel Thomson, but without relief.   The suffering becoming fearful, and life endangered, the old Dr. was sent for, and
a grain of Tartar Emetic relieved the stomach, and the boy
was asleep in an hour.   So I have had cases which were
speedily relieved by small doses of Sulphate of Magnesia, or
Iodide of Potassium—lead colic.   So we will find cases, requiring an absorbent like Charcoal, an Alkali, Ammonia,
Chloroform, Aromatics, even Podophyllin.   And again we
reach the conclusion that the pain was *not* the disease, not
even a reliable symptom.

Thus, in almost every case we are obliged to look beneath
the surface symptoms, and use our reasoning powers, compar-
ing the evidences of disease, and thus determining the exact
functional lesions.

Unless, and here is an important proviso, we have studied
this subject of *basic* symptoms ; then in a number of cases,
no matter what the disease, *the* remedy will be indicated by a
characteristic symptom.   In this I agree with some Homœopaths, as I agree that when a drug is thus clearly indicated,
it will probably be *the* remedy for the totality of the disease.
There is this difficulty here : in some cases there is no characteristic symptom, or if there is we have not learned to
know it, or have not learned *the* remedy.

But the cases given, though illustrating the necessity of
care in diagnosis, and the danger of falling into error, do not
otherwise bear upon our subject.   These cases are not obscure
if ordinary care is used, for the evidences of disease are un-
mistakable.   We have cases, however, in which great care is
necessary, and our diagnosis must be direct, differential, and
by exclusion.

Probably the shortest road to a correct idea of the methods

of diagnosis in the treatment of obscure cases, will be found in the following brief statement of the three methods above named :

1st. We have direct symptoms pointing to the seat, and the character of the disease. In simple cases these symptoms are clear and distinctive; in obscure cases, they are not, but they point the direction of investigation. If we have a single characteristic symptom, one that we have called *basic*, then of course our diagnosis is complete and the treatment definite.

2d. By *differential* diagnosis, we undertake to determine the location and character of disease by an analysis of the symptoms. Seeing which of them are common to all of the supposed affections—which are undeniably special to a certain part or function—until we have found one or more that locate the disease and determine its character.

3d. By *exclusion*, we give the entire body an examination, determining the functions that are *rightly* performed, excluding these, until finally we have localized the lesion and have determined its character.

There is hardly a disease so obscure but that it may be accurately determined in this way, if proper care is used. Necessarily we must know our Anatomy and Physiology, and the modern teachings of pathologists, then with caution and a right use of reason, we can hardly fail.

Now if we have determined such obscure disease, and we have had no experience and can find no treatment in our books, how shall we proceed? Very certainly as follows :

A drug is a remedy because it influences the part or function diseased. It is an indirect remedy when its influence is dependent upon the disturbance of some other part or function; it is a direct remedy, when its influence is directly upon the part.

Now we have determined the functions that are changed, and the part affected, we think of those remedies which are known to exert a more or less direct influence on the particular part or function; knowing the character of their action, and the want of the diseased body, we adapt the one to the other. If the case is one new to us, we may have to experiment, but the line of experiment will be a rational one, and likely to lead to good results.—*E. M. Journal, June,* 1872.

Epidemic or Endemic Constitution of Disease.

You have no doubt observed, that the diseases of some seasons, no matter how diverse in special characteristics, would have something in common, which something would be especially manifest in the treatment; that in some seasons Quinine would cure every thing, in others the sedatives would cure every thing, in others a remarkable benefit from Podophyllin, so that when you had once determined a good treatment, you would persist in it for all affections, with very little modification.

And this brings prominently before us the fact, for fact it is, that there is an endemic or epidemic constitution of disease, that should be well studied, and always regarded in treatment. Success or failure will very frequently depend upon this knowledge, and it is something that must be relearned every year.

It was a prominent doctrine of Rademacher and his followers, and he had remedies for three such constitutions. These were Iron, Copper, and the Nitrate of Soda. There was some truth in this—how much I don't know, for I have not had the opportunity to experiment, and, indeed, have not had time to give his works the examination they should have, as I read German slowly, and they have never been translated.

I believe, however, I have passed through one year, in which Iron was *the* remedy for almost every thing, and I think probably some of our old practitioners may recollect it, if they by chance had used Iron. The season commenced in December with a large number of cases of erysipelas, for which Iron was a specific, and for some fourteen months I prescribed Iron daily for almost every thing, with the most flattering results. I have experimented with Copper and Nitrate of Soda to but a limited extent.

Rademacher applied the principle to chronic disease. Grau-vogl says : "Our experience gained by this school is worthy of special consideration, 'that, in old *chronic* diseases, the previous epidemic constitution, always decides, first of all, upon the present indication of a remedy; hence, in every case which comes up for treatment, the time of its first ap-pearance should be learned, as far as possible, for by this, frequently, if the then epidemic curative remedy is known, the primary seat and the primary kind of the diseased pro-cess are known also, and this very remedy will still effect a cure, if a cure is yet possible, or, if the disease is not already succeeded by another disease of the first affected organ or blood, or if disease of another organ has not ensued. But, even in this latter case, that knowledge gives the point of de-parture for the whole chronic affection.'

"That is in gross what we see happen on a smaller scale, after strong or oft-repeated doses of long-acting remedies. First appear symptoms at the point of application, then of its reception in the blood; finally, the affections of the specifi-cally affected organs and systems in succession, and often at great intervals, as we have observed very distinctly with quicksilver, for instance. The only difference consists in this, that epidemic injurious influences, often after very many years, to the surprise of many, bring to view their *continued operation* as a token of the presence of their results under various forms of disease, while the continued operation of drugs is of proportionally shorter duration."—*E. M. Journal, June,* 1872.

CASES,

Illustrating Specific Medication.

The reader by this time will be impressed, that Specific Medication must be based upon specific diagnosis; that we prescribe medicines for pathological conditions, and not for names of disease; and that we will have success just in proportion as we learn the meaning of symptoms, and train our senses to close observation and an analysis of all the evidences of changes of function and structure.

True, we have to closely and carefully study our Materia Medica, and learn the influence of drugs upon the human body, this is an essential element of specific medication. But however well the physician may know his Materia Medica, if he can not recognize the evidences of disease, and the relation of remedies to definite conditions, he must fail in practice, or at least have only that success which comes from nature's efforts at cure, or by hap-hazard or indirect medication.

I confess it is not easy to learn this direct relation between disease and remedies. It is probably more difficult now than it will be years hence, when, having been more thoroughly studied it will be presented in a clearer light. Still it is our duty to make the most of what we have, trusting to time and careful observation to make up our present deficiencies.

I have thought that a report of cases illustrative of specific medication, would aid the reader, especially as they point out the symptoms or conditions of disease, that indicate special remedies. Many of these cases have been reported in the Eclectic Medical Journal, but I have given them the usual classification here.

Intermittent Fever.

We will take a series of cases illustrative of the treatment of intermittent fever. I confess, at the commencement, that I have not seen one case where others have seen fifty or one hundred, but I am very sure I have seen them with different eyes. It has been my fortune, however, to have seen, in the way of consultation, a large number of intractable cases, and one learns more from these than from the ordinary run of simple ones.

I may say, at the commencement, that while I value Quinine as a specific *against* the malarial poison (whatever it is) I do not regard it singly as a specific for the disease, or its common use as being good practice. I should prefer to dispense with it wholly in the treatment of periodic disease, than use it as badly as many do.

It is passing strange that doctors having eyes and a moderate amount of brains behind them, should persistently use Quinine in the most varying and opposite states of disease—in cases which have not a single thing in common but periodicity, and persist in its use when failure follows failure, and the only result of its administration is quinism—far worse than the original disease.

When a case of ague presents itself, we ask ourselves the question, is it *simple*, or is there functional or structural disease? If simple, the intermission is a state of perfect health, less a certain debility. If complicated, we wish to determine the exact condition of disease. If simple, we give Quinine at once; if complicated, we remove all functional and structural disease by appropriate remedies, and then, when simple, we give quinine if it is necessary. A large number of cases will not require it.

I administer Quinine differently from most physicians. The patient being properly prepared for its action, has a single dose of sufficient quantity to break the ague (grs. x. to grs. xv.), three hours before the expected chill. This is best taken dissolved in a small quantity of water by the aid of sulphuric acid. This may be called the big-dose plan. I have treated a few cases with a single dose of one-eighth of a grain, given at that period of the day when the patient is most himself—usually if the period of intermission is divided into three parts, the end of the first period will be the best time.

27

I will be glad if some of our readers, who have an abundance of cases, would try the small dose.

CASE I.—*Intermittent Fever—Inflammatory.*—F., æt. 41, a strong, robust man, has had ague for five months, contracted in the Wabash Valley. Has had it broken with Quinine, on an average, every two weeks. Has had a Thomsonian course of medicine, been freely purged with Podophyllin, and his liver tapped with Calomel and Blue Pill. His chill lasts from thirty minutes to two hours, and the fever severe, for six to ten hours, during which he suffers intensely. Is now quotidian.

Examination during the intermission shows : a dry, harsh skin ; a contracted tongue, with slight white coat down its centre, edges reddened ; some headache and backache at times, face flushed and eyes are bright and somewhat intolerant to a bright light; bowels constipated, (the patient claims they would never move without physic) ; urine diminished in quantity one-fourth, not changed in color. The pulse is 80, full and bounding. Temperature 100° scant.

Prescribed—℞ Tinct. Veratrum, gtts. xxx.; Tinct. Gelseminum, ℨj.; Water, ℥iv. ; a teaspoonful every hour until the pulse loses its full and bounding character, and the skin softens, then every three hours. Chlorform, gtts. xv. at the commencement of next chill. Acetate of Potash commenced on the third day, ℨij. daily. Hot foot-bath for thirty minutes every night on going to bed.

The chill and fever became lighter each succeeding day, and did not recur after the fifth day. If I had not been employing the remedies to determine their full influence in *curing* an ague, I should have given Quinia, grs. x. the third day, which, I have no doubt, would have broken the chill at once. The cure was a permanent one.

CASE II.—F., æt. 27, a brother of Case I. contracted the disease at the same time and place, and has pretty much the same experience, though Quinine has held the disease in check for longer periods. He is a spare man, and in appearance quite different from his brother, but the chill and fever are quite as severe. Ague is now tertian.

Examination during the intermission shows: a dry, harsh skin; pulse 86, *small and hard;* temperature 99½; urine scanty and high-colored (coloring matter biliverdin); tongue contracted and reddened; bowels regular.

Can not now take the smallest dose of Quinine without unpleasant head symptoms, and an increased severity in the fever.

Prescribed—℞ Tinct. Aconite, gtts. xx.; Tinct. Asclepias, ℨj.; Water, ℨiv. A teaspoonful every hour during the fever, every two hours in the intermission. Quinine inunction twice daily of: ℞ Quinia Sul., ℨij.; Lard, ℨij.; Oil of Anise, ℨss. M. Had two recurrences of ague after the treatment was commenced, but made an excellent recovery.

CASE III.—R., family of three, father, mother and child of three years. Had ague last year, and were cured with Quinine. (But like many cures with this drug, they were not entirely well.) Ague commenced this year in May, and for three months they have had it continuously. No means employed had done any good, except to break it on the father for one week. It is of the tertian type, but fortunately the sick day of one is the well day of the other. The sick day is a sick day in fact, as they keep the bed the whole day.

The father presents himself at the office on his well day. Examination shows—skin pallid and relaxed; pulse soft, open and easily compressed; temperature 99°; bowels tumid, irregular; hands and feet cold; eyes dull, pupils dilated; wants to sleep; tongue full, broad, with coating somewhat resembling that after eating milk. The others are represented as having the same symptoms.

Prescribed—℞ Tinct. Aconite, gtts. xv.; Tinct. Belladonna, gtts. xx.; Water, ℨiv.; a teaspoonful every two hours. Child one-fourth the quantity. Also Sulphite of Soda, grs. xx. three times a day.

Father reported in ten days that neither he nor the child had had a paroxysm of ague since, (the child did not take the Sulphite.) The mother had but two chills, but though better the disease was not arrested. Gave a single dose of Quinine, grs. x.; chills stopped, and thus far have not recurred. The entire family seems to be radically cured.

CASE IV.—W., Superintendent of Adams Express in the West, travels extensively in Southern Indiana, Illinois and Missouri; very strong and rugged, never had ague until August, 1870. Returned from Vincennes feeling very much depressed, had a slight chill, pain in head and back, intense muscular pain in right side extending from shoulder to foot. Eyesight impaired, and partial paralysis followed the subsidence of the pain; ague quotidian. These were the symptoms at each recurrence of the chills. I saw him soon after the second chill. The fever was very slight—notwithstanding the gravity of the other symptoms.

Prescribed—R Tinct. Aconite, gtts. x.; Tinct. Macrotys, gtts. xxx.; a teaspoonful every hour. The pain was speedily relieved by the prescription, and he slept well. Gave the succeeding forenoon, fifteen grains of Quinine in two doses. It had no more effect on the ague than so much water, but produced unpleasant head symptoms and deafness, which were persistent. Concluded to let Quinine alone, gave the first prescription only. There was a steady amendment, and the fourth day gave a single dose of Quinine, grs. x., and the disease was at an end for the time. Small doses of Quinine were taken as a prophylactic in his next trip.

Though the chills were stopped, the deafness continued, as did the slight paralysis. In September he had a recurrence of the disease in the same form. Concluded I would not use Quinine at all. Gave the Aconite and Macrotys the first day; then in addition—R Tinct. Nux Vomica, gtts. xx.; Water, ℥iv.; a teaspoonful every two hours (the remedies being alternated.) He had no recurrence of chill after the third day, and recovered his usual health rapidly. Has been in a malarial region this year—used no prophylactic—and has felt nothing of it.

The Nux Vomica was used in this case as a cerebro-spinal stimulant.

CASE V.—*Recent Ague.*—S. has had quotidian ague one week; been purged freely; and has had as much Quinine daily as his head would bear; feels badly, is discouraged, and concludes he will change doctors.

Characteristic symptoms—a broad, pallid tongue, coated with a white, pasty fur; breath fetid.

Prescribed—R Sulphite of Soda, grs. xx. every three hours. Had no more chills, and made a quick and permanent recovery.

This is a typical case, and some physicians have found all the cases of a season to take this character. Thus we had 127 cases reported by one physician in 1868, cured with Sulphite of Soda alone; Quinine failed almost uniformly.

Instead of depending wholly upon Sulphite of Soda, however, I would advise its use until this peculiar condition was rectified, and then give Quinine.

Common Salt has been successfully employed in the same class of cases in doses of grs. xx. every three hours during the intermission. A large number of cases, by different practitioners, were reported in one of our Southern exchanges, some twenty years ago.

CASE VI.—*Ague with Subsequent Typhoid Symptoms.*—Some fourteen years since I had to treat a very stubborn ague originating in the Little Miami bottoms. The cases would not yield to ordinary treatment; and in some, typhoid symptoms gradually developed, and patients died of what was at first an ordinary ague.

My first treatment was a complete failure, and it was only after I had seen a prescription of our old Quaker physician, Dr. William Judkins, that I had any success. It was very simple. Quinine, gr. j. every two hours during the intermission, with the free use of water acidulated with Nitro-Muri-atic Acid. The treatment was a complete success.

Characteristic symptoms—deep redness of mucous tissues, and dark coatings upon tongue; and to-day, with the same symptoms, I should use the same treatment.

CASE VII.—*Ague with Partial Congestion.*—F. has had ague for six weeks; has been twice broken with Quinine. Now Quinine has no influence, only to produce cerebral symptoms and increase the severity of the disease. Has been thoroughly purged with Podophyllin—worse. Has had two emetics—worse. Ague tertian.

His skin is sallow; yellowish discoloration about the mouth; complains of dull pain in right side under false ribs extending to shoulder, and occasional umbilical pains; en-largement of spleen, bowels irregular, stools clay colored; has frequent attacks of nausea; urine highly colored with bile; pulse in intermission 90, temperature 100°; has little appetite, and is very much debilitated.

Prescribed—℞ Tinct. Nux Vomica, gtts. x.; Water, ℥iv.; a teaspoonful every hour. The disease gives way slowly—patient had two chills after the medicine was commenced. The remedy was continued without change for two weeks, and the cure was permanent.

CASE VIII.—*Ague with Impaired Innervation.*—B. has had tertian ague for two weeks. There is nothing remarkable about the case, except the loss of energy and desire to do anything, and the fact that ordinary means do not reach it.

Pulse soft and open, 70 per minute; temperature 99°; skin relaxed and moist; tongue broad and sodden; bowels irregu-lar, stools semi-fluid with scybala; urine in large quantity, colorless.

Prescribed—℞ Strychnia, grs. 1-30th, every four hours dur-ing the intermission. Had no recurrence of chill, and made a good recovery.

I may say in this connection that the treatment of ague

with Strychnine is sometimes remarkably successful, and is again a complete failure. I think I have pointed out the Strychnine case, so that any of our readers may know it—but I would be very glad to have it confirmed by other observers.

Dr. Shultz, of Logansport, employs Strychnine, quite frequently, by hypodermic injection, and expresses himself pleased with its action.

CASE IX. — *Ague with Gastric Atony and Secretion of Mucus.*—Some thirteen years since I had to treat a number of cases of ague in river men. They had contracted the disease on the Lower Mississippi, Yazoo and Red River, and it was remarkably stubborn, some cases being continued from June to Mid-Winter, with temporary arrests from Quinine.

Three-fourths of them presented the following symptoms— tongue broad, heavily coated at base in the morning, bad taste in the mouth, weight and fullness in epigastrium, fetid breath, and unpleasant eructations after eating.

I treated every case with thorough emesis, (Compound Powder of Lobelia), repeated in some cases, and the use of a solution of Acetate of Potash, ℨiij. in twenty-four hours. No Quinine was used. The treatment was a decided success, but I obtained a reputation for giving nasty medicine that I never will get rid of. A few days since I met one of the patients, and he had to report how Dr. Scudder turned him inside out—but, says he, " I have been in the South every Summer since, and I have not had a shake."

Is this Specific Medicine too? Yea, verily, and very good practice it will be found in just such stubborn cases.

CASE X.—*Ague with Intestinal Torpor.*—I will not give a case, for any one of my readers can put his finger on one or more. Recollect that *constipation* is *not* the symptom; on the contrary the bowels will frequently move every day, yet the patient says the unpleasant feelings are never removed by it.

Characteristic symptoms—tongue full and coated from base to tip with a yellowish, pasty fur; bowels tumid.

Prescribe—Podophyllin thoroughly triturated, adding a small portion of Capsicum or Ginger, to free purgation. To be followed by Quinine when the system is in proper condition.

CASE XI.—*Ague treated with Arsenic.*—The first year of my practice I was poor, and found it difficult to make both ends meet. Late in the Fall I was applied to by a Southerner, who told me he had had ague for over a year; he had tried everything, and could get no relief. Could I help him? He had taken Quinine, Fowler's Solution, Salicine, and indeed all the common drugs.

I answered, yes, I'll cure you, (though I wasn't half as confident as I seemed).

Prescribed—Filled an ounce bottle one-fourth full of Homœopathic pellets, and dropped on them Fowler's Solution, gtts. v. Ordered ten of these every four hours. Only one chill afterwards, and made an excellent recovery.

The gentleman came to my office in about ten days, and after telling me that he thought he was well, and was going home, said, " Now, Doctor, I wont ask you what your bill is. There is $50 for the bottle of little pills, and you have my thanks in addition." That was the best money I ever made, for it enabled me to live until sufficient practice came.

In 1864 I had to treat three students who, coming from Missouri and Illinois, brought ague with them. During October and the first two weeks of November, they kept the disease partly in check by the use of Quinine and Podophyllin pills. But finally these failed, and the disease commenced to present typhoid symptoms, one of them being confined to his bed.

The symptoms were peculiar. There was no seeming loss of flesh, but the tissues seemed sodden, and expressionless. The tongue and other mucous tissues were tumid and bluish; a brownish fur gathered on the tongue, and sordes about the teeth; the bowels were loose, stools papescent; the chills not very severe, but the fever intense; pulse in intermissions, soft and fluent, during fever small and thready.

They were very bad cases, one was in a dangerous condition. They had taken the usual remedies, Quinine in full doses, as well as Strychnine; what should I give them? I decided at once to try the little pills. In a week the sickest one was at lectures.

Prof. Jones was told, and he was asked, "What the little pills were made of?" Of course he couldn't tell, and the very thought of *little pills* was an offence in his nostrils, and his remarks about "Dr. Scudder and his little jokers" were a standing subject for fun for many sessions.

Will the "little jokers" cure *all* cases of ague? Indeed they will not. I wish they would, for they are far pleasanter than Quinine. But they will cure *some* cases, and those are usually inveterate ones that Quinine won't reach.

"But!" and I imagine some one holds up his hands in holy horror, "that's giving Arsenic." That's a fact, so it is. I had forgotten that "ratsbane" was in the list of *tabooed* medicine. Got it mixed up with "hensbane" somehow. Very sorry, but these are facts, and we have need to know them.

CASE XII.—*Ague treated with Quinine Inunction.*—I reported my first case of ague cured by Quinine inunction some twelve years ago—and as it was a typical case, I may as well give it here.

A Mrs. Clark had suffered with ague for some five years— broken at times—but never free from its effects. It is now September, and she has had it since May with but one respite. Is very feeble, very sensitive, very nervous, and suffers severely. Can not take a grain of Quinine without cerebral symptoms; can not take the ordinary medicines in use, because they nauseate and are rejected by the stomach. Evidently a very bad case, and the young Doctor is at his wits' end to know what to do.

Had just been studying the action of remedies, and was at that time especially interested in cutaneous absorption, and concluded I would ask the skin to do the work of the stomach.

Ordered—℞ Quinia. Sul., ʒij.; Lard, ʒij.; to be thoroughly rubbed into the axillæ, and the anterior surface of abdomen. No more chills; made a slow, but excellent recovery.

I have used Quinine inunction in scores of cases since—not always with such positive results, but nearly always with benefit. In children it is a favorite remedy, especially in cases of *slow* infantile remittent. A physician of our school in Dayton, Dr. Kemp, tells me he has employed it in a large number of cases this year and last, and with the most flattering results.

CASE XIII.—*Ague cured by Cutaneous Absorption.*—John J. contracted ague during a visit West. Has been treated some weeks without benefit; has a horror of Quinine.

Used Ether Spray to chill a surface three inches in diameter over the epigastrium, and applied a Solution of Quinine. An application daily for a week, and the disease was permanently cured.

I have used Quinine in this way in a few cases, and in part of them with excellent results. Ether applied with a sponge, and evaporated by fanning, answers quite the same purpose as the spray apparatus. The Quinine is absorbed when reaction occurs, and it makes little difference to what part of the body it is applied, so the skin is thin.

CASE XIV.—*Ague cured with Boletus.*—M. has had ague off and on for two years. Quinine breaks the chill, but it returns within a week—and then for a time the drug has no influence. There is no special indication for any remedy.

Prescribed—℞ Tincture Boletus, ʒj.; Water, ʒiv.; a teaspoonful four times a day. Had no more chills, and the cure was radical.

I would be glad to have reports from physicians using Boletus, to show the *special* condition, if any, in which it is curative. For whilst curative in some, in others it exerts no more influence than water.

CASE XV.—*Chronic Ague.*—M., æt. 38, a river man, has been in the South-West for some six years, has had ague for the last three. Quinine will break it for a few days, but makes him feel so badly, that he dislikes to take it.

His skin is sallow, looks full and waxy, and has lost its natural elasticity; extremities are cold most of the time; urine in usual quantity, but of light specific gravity, 110 to 116; pulse is full, but shows want of power; bowels torpid; spleen much enlarged and tender; slight cough; tongue broad and furred white; appetite poor.

Prescribed—℞ Tinct. Veratrum, gtts. xx.; Water, ℥iv,; a teaspoonful every two hours. ℞ Acetate of Potash, ℨij. every twenty-four hours, in a considerable quantity of water. ℞ Tincture of Nux Vomica, gtts. ij. every morning in a glass of water.

Recovery was slow, but at the end of the month every vestige of ague had disappeared, and the patient was gaining flesh rapidly. The cure was permanent—has had no symptom of ague since, now three years.

The treatment of ague with Acetate of Potash was strongly recommended by Golding Bird in his work on Urinary Deposits, and will be found an excellent plan in some cases.

CASE XVI.—*Chronic Ague.*—C., æt. 26, has been a steamboatman on the Lower Mississippi for three years. Had ague the first year, which was cured with Quinine. Ague the second year was treated for some time without success, and was finally broken with Fowler's Solution in large doses—leaving him with the peculiar puffy condition of face and œdema of lower extremities, that so frequently follows this use of Arsenic. The third year the ague came on, and nothing would reach it, and he came here in September.

Skin is sallow, but looks like parchment and is tightly drawn to the tissues; pulse is small and frequent; urine is scant and high colored; bowels irregular, with occasional mucous diarrhœa; tongue looks lifeless, and is covered with a milky looking coat; appetite is poor; greasy eructations, and occasional vomiting of mucoid matter.

Prescribed—℞ Triturated Podophyllin, 1-100, grs. v.; Hydrastin, gr. ss. for a dose, three times a day. Quinia inunctions morning and night thoroughly. Every third day a thorough washing with soap and water.

Gained from the first day, and ceased taking medicine before the end of the third week. No recurrence of the disease.

The reader is ready to ask by this time, "Dr. Scudder, did you ever have any unsuccessful cases? Do you want us to believe that *your* medicine always works like a charm?" I answer, I have cases all the time in which my diagnosis is at fault—sometimes from carelessness, sometimes because I don't know. I would report these cases as well if I could see how a report of my want of care or want of skill could benefit the reader. I doubt not every one of my readers has a sufficient amount of that experience in his own practice, and need not go abroad for it.

What we want to know here, as in every other disease is—the *exact* condition of disease, and when we know this we can prescribe with certainty. Very certainly it requires something more than to say—" this is ague and I'll give Quinine;" that is further than I can go in Specific Medication.

CASE XVII.—*Chronic Ague cured with Iron.*—S., æt. 31, has suffered with ague for the past three years. It has been treated with Quinine, and he is now suffering from *quinism*, and at times the nervous symptoms are almost unbearable. The *special symptoms* are—a full *blue* tongue, and a cutaneous trouble showing the peculiar red glistening surface we see in some cases of erysipelas.

Prescribed—℞ Tinct. Muriate of Iron, ʒss; Simple Syrup and Glycerine, aa. ʒiv ; a teaspoonful four times a day. As a bath a weak solution of Sulphate of Iron. To wear red flannel. Made a good recovery, improving from the first, and has had nothing like ague for the six months past.

CASE XVIII.—*Chronic Ague cured with Nitric Acid.*—Dr. H., has suffered with ague for the past three years, which he has treated with Quinine—which will break the chills, but will not keep them off. Now Quinine irritates the nervous system, and the remedy is worse than the disease. Its manifestation now is in the form of periodic cephalalgia. *Special Symptoms* : A peculiar *violet* color upon a tongue moderately red. The lips and finger nails show the same violet haze.

Prescribed—℞ Nitric Acid, gtts. **xx** ; Water, Simple Syrup, aa. ℥ij ; a teaspoonful every three hours. The headaches recurred for three days, decreasing in severity, and there was complete and permanent recovery.

I have prescribed Nitric Acid in various forms of Chronic disease, when this peculiar symptom presented, with most satisfactory results, and would advise its trial.

Remittent Fever.

What we want to learn in regard to this disease might be divided into three parts. That, though the disease is called *bilious* fever, the liver has nothing to do with it. That, though classified as arising from vegetable malaria, for which Quinine is the specific, it is always best to treat the disease as if it were not so, until the fever, commencing to pass away, leaves the system in good condition for the kindly action of Quinine. And, lastly, there are cases, and seasons, where Quinine must be avoided, if we wish to have success, and not injure our patients. These points are pretty clearly set forth in the " revised edition " of my practice, to which the reader is referred.

CASE XIX.—*Simple Remittent Fever.*—There are localities in which the disease for several seasons will present a large number of *simple* cases. The patient has a well marked chill, followed by febrile action, and then a very decided remission, together occupying a period of twenty-four hours, and repeating the febrile exacerbation and remission in the same way, each succeeding day. You examine the patient carefully, and you find *nothing* but fever—no particular lesion of one part or function, more than another.

In these cases it is pretty safe to follow the rule of Prof. I.
G. Jones—Give a sufficient amount of Quinine during the
decline of the exacerbation and remission to stop the disease.
It will require from ten to fifteen grains. But if it fails the
first time, it is safer to prepare the system for its kindly action.

CASE XX.—*Simple Remittent Fever—killed by the Doctor.*
—James G., æt. 27, a strong, robust man, was attacked on a
Tuesday with a chill followed by high fever ; the next morning a decided remission, lasting an hour, then febrile action ;
no symptoms indicating complication, or danger. An Eclectic
was called, and commenced the treatment by the administration of Podophyllin pills to violent catharsis ; then Quinine
in divided doses ; then Podophyllin in *alterative* (?) doses (to
tap the liver) ; then more Quinine, alternated with Podophyllin.
Remainder of treatment—a nauseous diaphoretic stew, and
sweet Spirits of Nitre.

Saw the patient in consultation the next Tuesday morning.
Had furious delirium, requiring to be held on the bed ; skin
dry and harsh, pungent heat; mouth and tongue dry, tongue
furred, bleeding, almost black sordes upon teeth ; pulse 140,
small and hard ; eyes injected, pupils contracted, had not
slept for three days. Prognosis—death ; verdict—d—n the
doctor.

Did I ever do this thing? Probably not so grossly, though
it was rather from skepticism than good teaching that I
escaped. If I had followed instructions closely, I should
probably have ended some of my patients in the same way.

CASE XXI.—*Simple Remittent Fever Badly Treated.*—S.,
æt. 24, a robust, healthy woman, was attacked with remittent
fever, (Dr. called it bilious,) August 2d, From the history of
the case it was the simple form of the disease without complication. An active cathartic was prescribed, followed by alterative doses of a mercurial. Quinine was given in broken doses,
alternated with Dover's Powder, Spiritus Mindereri, and
Veratrum. The patient continued to get worse day by day,

and when I was called on the ninth day, was in the following
condition :

Tongue elongated and pointed, very dry, mucous tissues
dusky red, brown fur on center of tongue, and sordes on teeth;
pulse 130, small and sharp, temperature 106° in the evening,
103½° in the morning; delirium—a low muttering; skin harsh
and dry; urine scant and very red, bowels continuously loose
from the action of medicine, from the first.

Prescribed—R Dilute Muriatic Acid, Ʒss.; Simple Syrup,
Ʒjss.; a teaspoonful in water, every three hours. R Tinct.
Aconite, gtts. x.; Tinct. Gelseminum, Ʒss.; Water, Ʒiv.; a
teaspoonful every hour. A general sponge bath with soap
and water. After the second day Quinine inunction. A milk
diet.

No change was made in this treatment, and the patient was
convalescent in eight days after I took charge of her, making
seventeen days from the chill.

CASE XXII.—*Remittent Fever.*—O. B., æt. 17; was called
Aug 20th to take charge of the case, then in the fifteenth
day, the physician in attendance saying that the case must
prove fatal. Had the following history from parents and
physician :

Case not very severe at first; after sharp catharsis Quinine
was freely administered—patient much worse. More physic
and more Quinine, aided by Veratrum and Spiritus Mindereri—
still worse, Passing into the second week a diarrhœa became
a marked feature, for which was prescribed the usual astringents and Bismuth, but without any effect. Quinine still pushed.
Condition on fifteenth day :

Patient very feeble, lies on his back, has cough and difficult
respiration, has eaten nothing for three days, nor slept. Delirium constant, eyes bright and wild. Skin harsh and dry,
urine scanty. Diarrhœa a marked feature, actions passed in
bed whenever he coughs. Pulse 124, full but oppressed.
Temperature 103° morning, 106 evening. The tongue is not
much furred and is moist, but a dusky red. The patient is

very deaf, and has been so since the first week. Physical examination of the chest gives dullness on percussion over the lower lobe of both lungs, and moist blowing sounds over the entire chest.

Prescribed, for the diarrhœa—℞ Tinct. Aconite, gtts. x.; Tinct. Ipecac, gtts. xx.; Water, ℥iv.; a teaspoonful every hour. It did its work well, and we had no more trouble with diarrhœa after the fourth day, except for a brief period in the fourth week. The deep coloration of mucous membranes indicated an acid, and dilute Muriatic Acid was given in the usual way. Milk diet—the milk given hot four times a day, sometimes oftener.

For the delirium, I employed Prof. Howe's method—℞ Tinct. Aconite, ℥j.; Chloroform, ℥iij. M. To be applied freely to the nape of the neck, to control the cerebral disturbance and give sleep. To aid this, Gelseminum was given with the Aconite when there was no further need of the Ipecac; but this was only an aid, and we depended principally upon the local use of Aconite and Chloroform.

The disturbed condition of the brain was the result of Quinine, and it was the severest and the most persistent I ever saw. Though the patient was in good condition, and should have convalesced rapidly after the fourth week, we were obliged to use the local application of Aconite, for five weeks, making seven from the commencement, in order that he might sleep. Even now, thirteen weeks from first attack, his mind is not steady and he has the unpleasant roaring in his ears and deafness.

CASE XXIII.—*Simple Remittent Fever Badly Treated.*— O., a married woman, æt. 36, has been in feeble health for some years, though stout in body; was attacked with simple remittent fever, thought it was but a cold, and took on two successive days a patent pill to free purgation. Growing worse, a neighbor who dabbled in botanic medicine, proposed to give her a big sweat. This was effectually done, with a vapor bath, and an infusion of "boneset," and continued for

a day and night. Patient so much worse, that the writer was
sent for on the fifth day. Condition:—

Skin relaxed and bathed in perspiration, extremities cold,
trunk hot. Pulse 120°. Tongue moist, and covered with a
dirty fur, mucous membranes blueish. Bowels acted twice
during the day, stools large, papescent and light colored.
Urine moderately free. No appetite. Complained of sense
of fullness and also pain in the hypochondria and epigastrium.

Prescribed—℞ Tinct. Aconite, gtts. x.; Tinct. Belladonna,
gtts. xv,; Water, ℥iv.; a teaspoonful every two hours. ℞
Tinct. Nux Vomica, gtts x.; Water, ℥iv.; a teaspoonful
every two hours. Quinine inunction. Milk diet.

℞ Sulphurous Acid, ℥ss.; Simple Syrup, ℥jss.; a teaspoonful every three hours until the tongue cleaned.

The patient progressed favorably from the first, but it was
two weeks before fully convalescent.

Case XXIV.—*Remittent Fever presenting Typhoid Symptoms.*—Mrs. S., æt. 56. Has suffered for four months with
the unpleasant ague of this year, for which she has taken
different remedies, and prescriptions from two schools of medicine, but without benefit. Finally, on a visit to her son, the
fever assumed a remittent form, and she was confined to her
bed.

Symptoms—a marked chill with great prostration has been
occurring every day, for three days; before the ague was quotidian. Now her pulse is frequent, small, and oppressed,
skin dry and harsh, temperature 104° in afternoon, 102° in
morning, bowels loose, tongue moist and coated with a very
dirty brownish coat down the centre, sleeps but little, is very
feeble and depressed in spirits. There is a tendency to cold-
ness of the extremities—the feet will get cold if there is'not
a hot iron in bed, and the hands get cold when laid upon top
of the cover.

Prescribed—℞ Tinct. Aconite, gtts. x.; Tinct Belladonna,
gtts. x.; Water, ℥iv.; a teaspoonful every hour. On the
second day, in addition, ℞ Sulphurous Acid, ℥ss.; Simple

28

Sirup, ℥jss. M. S. A teaspoonful every three hours. On the fourth day, there was noticed a peculiar yellowness around the mouth, and the patient complained of umbilical pains, for which I gave : ℞ Tinct. Nux Vomica, gtts. x.; Water, ℥iv.; a teaspoonful every two hours alternated with the sedative.

The patient was free from fever by the seventh day, and made a sound and permanent recovery. Though two months have elapsed there has been no recurrence of the chills.

The need of Antiseptics in Typhoid Remittent (Typho-Malarial) Fever.—The cases of this year, 1871, have shown the marked importance of Antiseptics in these diseases. Not a single case of the seventeen that I treated, but was benefited by their use, and in some the need of the antiseptic was so marked that it alone would have given marked success.

We may study here seperately from the report of cases, four of the most important of these remedies—Sulphite of Soda Muriatic Acid, Sulphurous Acid, and Baptisia Tinctoria—the four fulfilling all the indications for an antiseptic treatment in all forms of disease. In the old routine of practice no one would have attempted to point out special indications for the use of either, but the writer would have said—here are four remedies that are likely to do good, try them in the order named until you find one to suit. I prefer, however, to select the remedy by certain specific symptoms, and not at random.

Sulphite of Soda—The indications for this antiseptic salt are : pallor of mucous membranes, usually fullness of tongue, and a pasty-white, or yellowish-white fur. We give it in doses of from five to twenty grains repeated every three hours.

Muriatic Acid.—We prescribe the acid where there is deep coloration of mucous tissues (not bright red), tongue contracted, coatings and sordes becoming brown as the disease advances. The usual prescription is : ℞ Dilute Muriatic Acid, ℥ss.; Simple Syrup, ℥jss. M. A teaspoonful every three hours, largely diluted with water.

Sulphurous Acid.—This is one of the feeblest of acids, and one of the most powerful of antiseptics. The indications for its use are—a moist tongue, neither pale nor deep-red, but showing a very unpleasant dirty clay-colored coat in the centre. The patient complains of fullness and weight in the epigastrium, an unpleasant taste in the mouth, and frequently has a disgust for food or drink. We prescribe it as follows: ℞ Sulphurous Acid, ℥ss.; Simple Syrup, ℥jss. M. A teaspoonful every three hours.

Baptisia Tinctoria.—There are none of our antiseptics that I value higher than this, and there is none which will give speedier relief if carefully prescribed. The indications for its use are clear (some of our readers may pronounce that *queer*)—fullness of mucous tissues, especially of throat, with bluish discoloration. Sometimes it is a bluish pallor, but more frequently it is deep bluish-red coloration. In the majority of cases, the breath will be fetid, fullness of epigastrium, tumid bowels, slimy offensive feces, and unpleasant odor both of urine and cutaneous excretion. I prefer to give it in infusion, ℥ss. to boiling water, ℥iv.; a teaspoonful every two or three hours.

The Use of Belladonna.—In the treatment of the fevers this year, we have found that Belladonna was a very important remedy. Associated with Aconite, it would cure ague, when Quinine had failed, and in many cases of this *typho-malarial* fever, its beneficial influence was marked, both upon the nervous system and upon the circulation.

Now what is the *specific* indication for Belladonna? It is clearly this—an enfeebled capillary circulation. If this lesion is principally of the brain, we have impaired innervation—dullness, somnolence, coma; if of the spinal cord—impaired respiration, urination, defecation, but more markedly a tendency to congestion of the thoracic and abdominal viscera.

How do I know that Belladonna stimulates the capillary circulation? I knew it nearly or quite ten years ago through Brown-Sequard's eyes—he *saw* the dilated capillaries contract under the general influence of Belladonna in small doses, as plainly as I see my hand carrying the pen over this paper. And I have seen it ever since, in the subsidence of symptoms caused by capillary congestion, where the remedy is properly administered.

CASE XXV.—*Remittent Fever.*—J. H., æt. 28, has been feeling badly for the past ten days, and has been confined to the house for three days. Has had two chills, with constant fever since—but slight morning remission. Says he feels very sick, can not sleep, and complains of a sense of weight and oppression in epigastrium, and indeed the entire abdomen.

The pulse is 120, full but not hard, temperature $104\frac{1}{4}°$ evening, 102° morning, skin hot but not very dry, urine scanty and odor very unpleasant, bowels constipated. The mucous membranes of the mouth markedly *pallid*, tongue full and coated with a thick white fur.

Prescribed—Add Bicarbonate of Soda to Water to make a pleasant drink, to be taken *ad libitum.* ℞ Tinct. Aconite, Tinct. Belladonna, aa. gtts. x.; Water, ℨiv.; a teaspoonful every hour. A soda bath once daily. Milk diet. Was markedly improved the first twelve hours, sleeping at night, and was convalescent the sixth day of treatment.

In this case the indication for the use of the Salt of Soda was very marked, hence this became the principal element of a successful treatment; and though the case was a severe one it rapidly yielded to these simple means.

CASE XXVI.—*Remittent Fever.*—Mrs. S., æt. 32, has been suffering with "bilious fever" for six days, and concludes to change physicians. Presents no very unfavorable symptoms, though the friends claim that all the medicine she has taken has made her worse.

Symptoms—skin dry and harsh; evening temperature 106°; features sharpened, eyes bright and intolerant of light, is restless and uneasy, and does not sleep well; urine scanty and high colored; has been freely purged, but bowels still constipated; pulse hard, 120; mouth dry, tongue contracted and beginning to fissure, brownish sordes in fissures and forming on teeth; color of mucous membranes *deep-red*; can not take food or medicine without unpleasant sensations in the stomach, and nausea.

Prescribed—℞ Dilute Muriatic Acid, ℥ss.; Simple Sirup, ℥jss. M. A teaspoonful every three hours—added to water to form a pleasant acid drink. ℞ Tincture Aconite, gtts. x.; Tincture Gelseminum, gtts. xx.; Water, ℥iv.; a teaspoonful every hour. An acid bath. Milk diet. Was convalescent the fourteenth day of the disease, the eighth of this treatment.

Case XXVII.—*Remittent Fever.*—A., æt 36, a railroad laborer, has been employed in the Miami bottoms, and came home very sick—has been feeling badly for a week.

Complains of severe pain in back and limbs, muscles stiff, feel as if bruised—has had it from the commencement, chill two days since, high fever following, with morning remissions. Pulse 110, full and hard; skin hot and dry, temperature 105° evening; tongue natural in size and color, dry, with a clear white coat; bowels constipated; urine scanty and high-colored.

Prescribed—℞ Tinct. Veratrum, gtts. xx.; Tinct. Aconite, gtts. x.; Tinct. Macrotys, gtts. xxx.; Water, ℥iv.; a teaspoonful every hour. Alkaline sponge bath. Milk diet. Marked relief from pain in twelve hours, and the fever declining to the fourth morning of treatment, found the skin soft, pulse soft and full, tongue moist and cleaning—gave two doses of Quinine, grs. iv., at intervals of three hours, and the fever was arrested.

Case XXVIII.—*Remittent Fever.*—W. R. has been suffering from fever for four days, medicating himself, aided by his family. Has taken *at* an emetic, has taken freely of Podophyllin pills, and on two successive days has had Quinine. Feels very badly, and is quite sick.

Symptoms—pulse 110, small and oppressed; skin hot and dry; bowels loose from medicine; urine scanty but colored with bile; stomach irritable, with nausea; has an uneasy

sensation and fullness in hypochondria, with occasional umbilical pain; cough beginning to develop itself unpleasantly;
face is sallow, and yellowness is especially marked about the
mouth.

Prescribed—℞ Tinct. Aconite, Tinct. Ipecac, aa. gtts. x.;
Water, ℥iv.; a teaspoonful every two hours. ℞ Tinct. Nux
Vomica, gtts. x.; Water, ℥iv.; a teaspoonful every two hours,
alternate. A wet pack over epigastrium. Milk diet. Was
free from fever the fourth day of treatment.

CASE XXIX.—*Remittent Fever, with Suppression of the
Menses.*—Mrs. J. has been feeling badly for ten days, has had
the chills, but the last two days the fever is constant. It is
now time for the menstrual period.

Commenced treatment with the use of Veratrum and
Aconite, the bath, hot foot-bath, a saline purgative, afterwards a saline diuretic, and continued in this way for five
days, patient getting worse. Gave the sedative more freely,
and in morning remission used the hot foot-bath and Asclepias, and followed with Quinine. Patient grew worse rapidly
after the Quinine was given, being very restless, some delirium,
and the stomach irritable. Treatment has now occupied
seven days—without any benefit—and came to the conclusion
that I had better study the case if my patient is to live.

A few questions and a little thought point out the menstrual
derangement as an important element of the disease. Prescribe—℞ Tinct. Pulsatilla, gtts. x.; Tinct. Macrotys, gtts.
xx.; Water, ℥iv.; a teaspoonful every two hours—alternated
with: ℞ Tinct. Aconite, gtts. x.; Water, ℥iv.; a teaspoonful
every two hours. A warm pack to lower abdomen. Patient
was decidedly better in twelve hours, and the fever declined
rapidly, though the menstrual discharge did not commence
until the third day after this change of treatment, and when
patient was nearly freed from fever.

Infantile Remittent Fever.

If there is any one thing more than another that I prize, it is the name of being a "good doctor for children." And if there is any one thing more than another that the Old-School practice deserves deepest damnation for, it is their miserable life-destroying practice in the diseases of childhood. I shudder as I look back on my earlier experience in medicine and recall the many cases where 1 have seen the innocents tortured, as only doctors can torture, and I wonder that people can believe in special providences, when such things were permitted.

Give the little sufferer from the many ills of childhood, good nursing, cleanliness, proper food and rest, and you will have a treatment that at least does not violate the seventh commandment. Supplement this with the mild but direct remedies of our practice, and you relieve disease of half its suffering, shorten its duration, and save life.

CASE XXX. — *Typical Infantile Remittent.* — Pulse 120; temperature 104° in exacerbation; skin dry; tongue slightly reddened and covered with a whitish fur; restless and uneasy during the exacerbations. Remissions in the fever vary in different cases, sometimes but one, at others three, four or more, in twenty-four hours. Nothing but fever.

Prescribe—℞ Tinct. Aconite, gtts. v.; Water, ℥iv.; a teaspoonful every hour. Bath once or twice daily. No other medicine.

CASE XXXI. — *Infantile Remittent, with Irritation and Determination of Blood to the Brain.* — A., æt. twenty-one months, was attacked with simple fever, and the nearest physician was called, prescribing the usual cathartic and Sweet Spirits Nitre. The second day the child was very restless, its face flushed, the stomach irritable, fever high, and in the afternoon had a convulsion. Having been the family physician, was now sent for. Symptoms—face flushed, eyes bright, pupils contracted, skin hot and dry, pulse 146, small and sharp, unconscious, moving head from side to side, involuntary movements of hands and feet—bad case.

Prescribed—℞ Tinct. Aconite, gtts. v.; Tinct. Gelseminum, gtts. xx.; Water, ℥iv.; a teaspoonful every thirty minutes, until the fever is reduced and head relieved. Towel wrung out of cold water over stomach and abdomen.

Had relief and sleep by 4 o'clock next morning. Reduced the proportion of Gelseminum to gtts. x., continuing every hour, and the fever ceased the fifth day.

CASE XXXII.—*Infantile Remittent Fever, with Cerebral Congestion.*—Annie L., æt. three years, was attacked with fever August 4th. The mother noticed that she was very dull, and slept with her eyes partly open. Had a Homœopathic case in the house, and gave her Aconite. The night passed, and the child was worse, and I was sent for, seeing her about noon. The symptoms now were very distinct—the child was sleeping with its eyes half open, its face expressionless, the eyes dull, pupils dilated; the skin was hot and dry, pulse 130, symptoms of convulsions.

Prescribed—℞ Tinct. Aconite, gtts. v.; Tinct. Belladonna, gtts. x.; Water, ℥iv.; a teaspoonful every hour.

The coma gradually passed off, the fever was reduced, and the next morning the child was comparatively comfortable and was discharged on the 9th.

CASE XXXIII.—*Infantile Remittent Fever, with Intestinal Irritation.*—W., æt. 28 months, was attacked with fever Sept. 20th. Called the next day, found febrile action high, stomach irritable, and some three or four greenish watery discharges from the bowels.

Prescribed—℞ Tinct. Aconite, gtts. iij.; Tinct. Ipecac, gtts. x ; Water, half a teaspoonful every thirty minutes until the stomach is relieved, then a teaspoonful every hour. Convalescent on the morning of the 24th.

Case XXXIV.—*Infantile Remittent cured with Nux Vomica.*—Pat R., æt. 5, has been sick for a week past. Has had the city physician, who gave Quinine, which stopped the fever, and the patient was discharged. Fever returned, with nausea and vomiting, and I was sent for.

Symptoms—Pulse 120; skin sallow and dirty, yellowish around the mouth; complains of pain in the abdomen; tongue broad, moist, and coated with a dirty fur.

Prescribed—R Tinct. Nux Vomica, gtts. iij.; Water, ℥iv.; give half a teaspoonful every fifteen minutes until the vomiting ceases, then a teaspoonful every hour. Better the next morning, has not vomited since the evening before; pulse 90; tongue showing a tendency to clean; rested well the after part of the night. Improved steadily, and was convalescent on the sixth day, no other medicine being given.

Case XXXV.—*Infantile Remittent—Malarial.*—Jessie C., æt. 4 years, was attacked with remittent fever September 3d. Called to see her on the morning of the 4th, presented the usual febrile symptoms, with some irritation of the brain.

Prescribed—R Tinct. Aconite, gtts. v.; Tinct. Gelseminum, gtts. xx.; Water, ℥iv.; a teaspoonful every hour; with the usual bathing and nursing. There was relief from the nervous irritation, and some mitigation of fever, but the disease continued. Continued the same treatment to the 9th, when I concluded, as the child had been on a visit to a malarial region, to give Quinine, grs. iij. There was no more fever.

Case XXXVI.—*Infantile Remittent — Malarial.*—Byrd Scudder, æt. 3, a stout, active boy, was playing for hours on a yellow clay bank, one of the hottest days in June. The next day he had a chill, and following this a very high fever, with but slight remissions. Irritation of the nervous system, and strong symptoms of convulsions. One of the sickest children I ever saw.

Prescribed — R Tinct. Aconite, gtts. v.; Tinct. Gelseminum, gtts. xx.; Water, ℥iv.; a teaspoonful every hour. The

29

fever was but little influenced by the medicine, though the
nervous system was relieved, and continued for thirty-six
hours. Now there was a complete intermission of eight
hours, when it recommenced as severe as before, and continued forty-eight hours, with a second intermission. As he
had an utter disgust for nasty medicine (which, by the by, he
inherited from his father) I withheld Quinine, and continued
the febrifuge. The fever came up as before, and continued
again for thirty-six hours, and again an intermission but not
as complete. Was now ready to give Quinine, and administered three grains, and ordered it by inunction. No more
fever.

I might report a score of cases in which I have administered Quinine early, with the result of increasing the disease.
In malarial districts it becomes a part of the treatment of
every case; in some being specific to the disease without
other treatment, but in the majority the system should be
prepared for its use as heretofore named. In our city, malarial disease is the exception, and we don't use Quinine so frequently or so freely.

Continued Fever.

CASE XXXVII.—*Continued Fever. Experiment with Quinine.*—Charles W., æt. 23, had a chill November 20, had
been feeling badly for some two weeks. When called on the
24th found the usual symptoms of continued fever, with no
special indication for treatment other than this.

Prescribed—℞ Tinct. Veratrum, gtts. xx.; Tinct. Aconite,
gtts. x.; Water, ℥iv.; a teaspoonful every hour. Use the
bath once daily. As is common with these remedies there
was slight abatement of the fever from day to day, until on
the 27th it seemed as if but little more would give convalescence. The skin was soft, pulse soft and open, tongue moist,
the condition for Quinine. Ordered three grains every two
hours for four doses. The first influence seemed that desired—
the pulse gained fullness and came down to 70, and the sur-

face became moist, but following this there was slight chill, and the fever came up rapidly. The next day the patient was far worse than he had been, and required constant and careful attention up to the twenty-fourth of the disease.

From this, and some other experience of a similar kind, I learned not to give Quinine in large doses in continued fever.

CASE XXXVIII.—*Continued Fever.*—B——, æt. 36, has been feeling badly for ten days. Yesterday had a slight chill in the morning, and again in the afternoon, fever at night, gradually increasing. Has the usual symptoms of common continued fever, which is now prevailing, but without any special indication for remedies, other than this. Pulse full and hard, 110; temperature on the third day 103° morning, 105½° evening.

Prescribed—℞ Tinct. Veratrum, gtts. xxx.; Water, ℥iv.; a teaspoonful every hour. The usual bathing and good nursing. No influence upon the fever seemingly, until the morning of the fifth day, though the patient was relieved of suffering. Now the fever seems inclined to yield, pulse 84 in the morning and open, temperature 101°; afternoon pulse 96, temperature 102¼°. Prescribed—℞ Tinct. Veratrum, gtts. xx.; Tinct. Aconite, gtts. x.; Tinct. Asclepias, ʒj.; Water, ℥iv. 6th day. Morning, pulse 80, temperature a fraction less than 100°; evening, pulse 90, temperature, 102°. Added Solution of Acetate of Potash. 7th day. Morning, pulse 80, temperature 100¼°; evening pulse 96, temperature 102°. Tongue is moist and shows a tendency to clean; skin is soft and occasionally moist. Continued in this way with but little change to the fourteenth day, when the fever ceased, and the patient convalesced rapidly.

In some cases, presenting like symptoms, I have added small doses of Quinine to the treatment with the effect of arresting the fever sooner.

CASE XXXIX.—*Continued Fever. Special Indications for Treatment.*—I will next present my own case, as reported February, 1865. Treatment by Prof. King:

"Fortunately for me the type of continued fever changed about the middle of December; whereas previously every case was attended by disease of Peyer's glands and diarrhœa, (typhoid), after this time it was common continued fever without the least tendency to enteric disease. The first conclusion forced upon me was that a physician is incompetent to prescribe for himself; as the disease came upon me, and assumed its most severe form without my being aware of what was the matter.

"It was attended for the first week with very severe pain in the back, limbs, joints, etc., so much so that I supposed at first it was rheumatic fever. The simple means employed at first—hot foot bath, spirit vapor-bath and diaphoretics—having failed, on the fourth day, I resolved to try the virtues of Quinine to stop the fever, and to relieve the pain, and accordingly took fourteen grains in six hours, and repeated it the succeeding day. It did seem to arrest all the febrile symptoms, but it was followed by great prostration and exhaustion of the nervous system. Having had enough of my own treatment, Prof. King was called to prescribe, and it is the means he used that I wish to notice.

"My condition may be briefly described as follows: Tongue broad, and thickly coated with a white fur, bowels constipated, a feeling of weight and dullness in the basilar and posterior portions of the head, pain in the lower part of the back, and wandering pain in the limbs. Sleeplessness and nervous excitement, pulse 130, soft, small and very feeble.

"The doctor claimed that the white tongue indicated acidity, not only of the stomach, but an undue amount in the blood. To relieve this, he ordered Bicarbonate of Soda, a teaspoonful to a tumbler of water: a swallow to be taken every few minutes during the day. Its taste was very pleasant to me, and its influence agreeable, and though I had not the slightest feeling of acidity of the stomach, I am satisfied that it supplied a material that was deficient.

"To assist in removing the nervous prostration, and to relieve the pain, my back and limbs were to be rubbed morning and night with brandy, holding in solution five grains of Quinine to the ounce; one ounce to be used for a bath. Of all the remedies I ever employed none had so speedy and pleasant an effect as this, and I continue it at the present time. I consider it an item worth recollecting.

" Internally I was given a combination of half a grain of Quinine with four grains of diaphoretic powder, repeated every four hours. Under this treatment my pulse came down, I obtained refreshing sleep, and by the third day, secretion from the skin and kidneys was established. To move my bowels, I was ordered one grain of Leptandrin, triturated with white sugar, three times a day; the doctor claiming that as soon as the liver was stimulated to action my bowels would move. Having had no operation for four days, the first three powders moved the bowels kindly; the first instance in which I was ever satisfied that the remedy would prove cathartic.

"Altogether, the treatment was a success, and I am satisfied that certain parts of it are well worthy of trial. Convalescence has been slow, and I am still very feeble, but gaining ground every day. I have proven on my own person what I had long been convinced of, that the use of tonics and stimulants, in a majority of cases of continued fever, does not facilitate convalescence, but that in many cases their action is the reverse of that desired.

CASE XL.—*Continued Fever. Requires an Alkali.*—Jas. L—— was attacked Dec. 4th with chill, pain in head and back and general malaise; had been feeling badly for some days. Next day was better, but in the evening had a second chill. Third day started to business, but felt so badly returned home by 10 o'clock, suffering from chills, and went to bed; fever came up in the afternoon, and he passed a restless night.

Called on the morning of the 4th. Pulse 110, small and hard, temperature 103½°. Tongue moist, broad, thick, pallid, and covered with a white pasty coat; breath has a peculiar sweet, mawkish odor.

Prescribed—Bicarbonate of Soda in water as a drink *ad libitum.* ℞ Tinct. Aconite, gtts. x.; Water, ℨiv.; a teaspoonful every hour. A Soda water bath. Amendment from the first, and was convalescent by the seventh day of treatment.

The joke was, there was a Regular physician in the house—a relation, who claimed that there was no salvation for the patient except by the use of Calomel or Blue-pill; insisting that the peculiar appearance of the tongue was a strong indication for mercurials.

CASE XLI.—*Continued Fever.—Requires an Acid.*—John B——, æt. 41, has been sick for two weeks with the prevailing fever, under regular treatment. Friends conclude to change treatment, and the attending physician is discharged, and I am called.

Condition—Has been delirious for the past four days, and sleeps but very little. The face is flushed and dusky, eyes injected. The skin is dry and harsh, the urine scanty, the bowels freely acted upon by physic, are now irritable, abdomen tender. Pulse 130; temperature 107° in the evening. The tongue is *dark red*, contracted, and covered with a brownish fur, sordes on the teeth.

Prescribed—℞ Dilute Muriatic Acid, ℨss.; Simple Syrup, ℨjss.; add to water to make a pleasant drink, and give *ad libitum.* Use an acid bath twice daily. ℞ Quinia Sul., ℨij.; Dilute Muriatic Acid, ℨiv.; a tablespoonful to a pint of water, for a bath. Milk diet.

No change was made in the treatment, the patient improving steadily to convalescence on the twenty-third day from the commencement of disease.

I report a typical case, in which nothing but an acid was used—it might be called a test case. Though the indications for acids are so pronounced that they form the basis of a good treatment, yet we employ various means in addition, as they may be indicated.

It might be said that twenty-one days being the natural duration of such a fever, the acid was a mere placebo. But I answer, there was relief from the more urgent symptoms within forty-eight hours, and this alone was worth working for, without reference to the duration of the disease.

CASE XLII. — *Continued Fever, with Disease of Peyer's Glands—Typhoid Fever.*—R——, æt. 29, now in the second week of a typhoid fever, has a sudden accession of diarrhœa, with abdominal tenderness, and an increase of typhomania. The discharges are very peculiar, frothy, illy concocted, and have a very unpleasant cadaveric odor. The tongue is moist, and shows a very dirty coat. The symptoms are very grave.

Prescribe—℞ Sulphurous Acid, Simple Sirup, aa. Зj.; a teaspoonful every three hours. ℞ Tinct. Aconite, gtts. x.; Tinct. Ipecac, gtts. xx.; Water, Зiv.; a teaspoonful every hour for two hours, the third hour the acid; Quinine inunction to abdomen. Must maintain the recumbent position.

The treatment served the purpose, the diarrhœa was checked, and by the third day the patient was taking his milk kindly, and convalesced the fourth week.

CASE XLIII. — *Continued Fever, with Disease of Peyer's Glands—Typhoid.*—O. M——, æt. 18, is in the third week of typhoid fever with Homœopathic practice, and is "given up" as incurable.

Condition.—Lies on the back continually, picks at the bed clothes, muttering delirium, face and eyes congested. Tongue, fauces and pharynx swollen, and of a deep purplish color, dark brown, nasty coat on tongue, bowels tympanitic, stools dark and excessively fetid, pulse 130, without strength, temperature 105½ evening.

Prescribed—℞ Baptisia Tinctoria in infusion, a teaspoonful every two hours, also wash the mouth with it. ℞ Tinct. Aconite, gtts. v.; Tinct. Belladonna, gtts. x.; Water, Зiv.; a teaspoonful every two hours. Use an acid bath (muriatic) with Quinine. On the third day of this treatment there was decided improvement, the diarrhœa checked. Now added

Muriatic Acid internally, and continued to convalescence on the twenty-sixth day of the disease.

CASE XLIV.—*Continued Fever, Typhoid, with Retention of Urine.*—M. C—— is in the second week of typhoid fever. The typhomania has been a marked feature, and is now sinking to a muttering delirium. Muscular feebleness has been especially marked, and now the patient lies on the back and slips toward the foot of the bed. On the morning of the thirteenth day found retention of urine, and difficulty in respiration.

There has been seemingly an indication for an acid treatment in the deep-red of the tongue and mucous membranes. The feeble pulse and tendency to congestion seemed to call for Aconite and Belladonna. But the treatment thus far has been a failure, and unless something more is done the patient will die.

Drew off the urine with catheter, and prescribed: ℞ Solution of Strychnia, ʒj.; Liquor Bismuth, ℥iv.; a teaspoonful every three hours. Add Bicarbonate of Potash to water, so that it will be pleasant to take and use as a drink; a weak lye as a bath once daily. There was marked improvement within twenty-four hours, and the patient convalesced, without change of remedies.

Here was one of those rare cases in which, though there was an alkaline condition, there was a want of Potash as shown by the extreme muscular feebleness, and the salt of Potash became a true restorative; whilst Strychnia increased innervation from the spinal cord and sympathetic, and was just what was needed to increase the strength of the circulation and respiratory movement.

Smallpox.

There are three features in this disease that demand particular attention: 1, The disease is exhaustive; 2, there is impairment of the function of the skin; 3, there is the tendency to blood poisoning—sepsis. If we neglect to provide against these, in severe cases we may have death result from any one of the three.

We say, therefore: That we must keep the stomach and intestinal canal in good condition for the reception of food, and for its digestion; and see that the patient has it frequently and in proper form. That under no circumstances must the eruption be determined to the skin so as to impair its function to the amount of five-sevenths. That in all cases the patient be protected against blood poisoning, and that the proper antiseptics be continuously used.

I recognize the fact that the same pathological laws govern this as other fevers, and that therapeutic means are quite as definite and certain. As is the frequency of pulse and increase of temperature, so is the severity of the disease— marked by arrested secretion, impaired digestion, derangement of the nervous system, blood-poisoning, and extent of eruption. As we follow the ordinary indications in the treatment of a fever—bring down the pulse, lessen the temperature, establish secretion, and support the strength, the disease becomes mild, and the eruption discrete.

I propose, therefore, the use of the proper sedatives, the bath, alkaline diuretics, and occasional laxatives, and the proper antiseptics, with good feeding, as a rational treatment of smallpox. I claim that with this treatment, the disease may not only be rendered much milder, but in some cases may be aborted, as I have conclusively proven in my practice.

The ordinary treatment of this disease is radically wrong, and is in part the cause of its fatality. As is well known, it consists in the frequent and continuous use of purgatives, and stimulant means to determine the eruption to the skin. The one impairs the action of the intestinal canal, the other the function of the skin. Both are absolutely prohibited in my treatment, under all circumstances. I may also say that the patient can not bear the use of the large doses of Veratrum named in the books, and a fatal result may be readily obtained with this.

CASE XLV.—M——, a member of the present class was attacked in the following way: Had suffered for three days with a sense of depression, aching in back and limbs, and loss of appetite. Then a well marked chill, followed by high fever.

When I was called, found the pulse full and hard, 120 per per minute; skin dry and hot, face flushed, eyes bright, tongue *pallid* and coated from base to tip with a very nasty white coat; throat much swollen, showing a bluish pallor; is very restless and can not sleep, no appetite.

Ordered—Add Bicarbonate of Soda to water to make a pleasant drink, and give him all he wishes. R Tinct. Veratrum, gtts. x.; Tinct Gelseminum, gtts. xx.; Water, ℥iv.; a teaspoonful every hour.

Found the next morning that he had taken the Soda water by the pint, and that it had passed off freely by the bowels. The *pallor* of mucous membranes was replaced by deep redness, the pulse was 90; patient better in every respect. Continued the sedative, and ordered for the day diluted Muriatic Acid as a drink. The third day from chill, the eruption commenced making its appearance, and the next day covered the body as thickly as I ever saw it in the severest confluent form of the disease.

On the fourth day, Sulphurous Acid was given as the antiseptic, the Veratrum being continued. And this was the treatment so long as any was needed. The eruption in the throat was as severe as ever I witnessed it, and the discharge from the mouth excessive. The eruption on the face did not fill, neither did it on many parts of the body. Medicine was suspended the eighth day.

CASE XLVI.—*Confluent Smallpox.*—L. S., confluent small-pox of severest type. Throat symptoms very marked, and secretion of mouth and throat abundant and offensive. The odor of smallpox is so strong that it permeates the entire house, and is almost unendurable in the room. It is now the fifth day from the chill; the patient has been in the hands of another physician, and doctors are changed because, it is im-possible for him to take medicine. Has had purgatives every day and various nasty potions. The one favorable feature is— the eruption is out, though the skin is dusky. Find it abso-lutely impossible for patient to take medicine or food; the stomach would not tolerate it, and the patient can not swallow it.

Treatment.—Have the stove taken out of the room, and a fire built in the open fireplace; one window being opened to give free ingress of air. The room thoroughly cleaned, the patient washed, and clothing of person and bed changed. Let the mouth and throat be washed with salt water suffi-ciently often to free it from the secretions, and give small por-tions of a weak salt water as a drink. Burn a small portion of Sulphur by the bedside every three hours. Wash the patient thoroughly with soap and water every day.

On the second day the patient was able to take food, and from the third day on he took corn meal gruel and milk freely. The unpleasant odor had nearly disappeared the third day, and the septic symptoms rapidly abated. The patient made a good convalescence in the usual time, no medicine having been given.

I give this as a marked example of the benefit to be ob-tained from antiseptic treatment. The agent here was Sul-phurous Acid, set free by burning Sulphur. It influenced the contagion directly, and its inhalation was quite as efficient in checking the blood poisoning as if it had been given by mouth.

CASE XLVII.—*Confluent Smallpox.*—N., æt. 5, never vac-cinated, has had severe fever four days, with the pain, fullness of skin, furred symptoms and peculiar odor that indicate smallpox. The skin is flushed and dusky, the patient comatose.

Prescribed—℞ Tinct. Aconite gtt. v.: Tinct. Belladonna, gtt. v. Water ℥iv.: a teaspoonful every hour.

In twelve hours the nervous system was freed, the patient conscious, and the eruption coming out nicely. Sulphite of Soda, the antiseptic remedial, was prescribed in addition, and with cleanliness, the use of the bath, and fluid food, the patient convalesced at the usual time.

Case XLVIII.—*Confluent Smallpox.*—C. is now in the seventh day of the disease, eruption out and filling. Pulse is small and hard, 120 beats per minute, temperature 106°. Skin dusky, eruption dark colored, mouth dry, tongue almost black, sordes on teeth, has been delirious since the third day.

Prescribed—℞ Tinct. Muriatic Acid ℥ss.: Simple Syrup, ℥ss.: a teaspoonful every two hours in his drink. ℞ Tinct. Aconite gtt. xx.: Tinct. Lobelia gtt. xx.: Water, ℥iv.: a teaspoonful every hour. Fluid food with a small portion of brandy every three hours and Quinine Injection to the abdomen.

Patient pulled through it, and made a good convalescence.

Measles.

If I was writing for the profession at large, I would probably give my treatment with the medicines—and leave the case to nature, aided by such simple aids as are given in most households. For here it is very serious, the mortality is in proportion to the amount of medication, and it is much better to dispense with the physician when there is real need for aid than have the ordinary routine of treatment.

Case XLIX.—*Rubeola.*—Four children of Mr. —— were attacked with measles in January. Two of them had it quite severely, the temperature at one marking 104°. There was more than the usual bronchial irritation in all, and in one it was very severe.

In two of the cases there was oppression of the nervous system, and a tendency to sleep all the time before the eruption. For these I prescribed: ℞ Tinct. Aconite, gtts. v.; Tinct. Belladonna, gtts. viij.; Water, ℥iv.; for a girl of eight years, a teaspoonful every hour; for a child of four, half a teaspoonful every hour. The others had: ℞ Tinct. Aconite, gtts. v.; Tinct. Ipecac, gtts. xv.; Water, ℥iv.; a teaspoonful every hour, until the fever abates; and this was given to the first two when the eruption had appeared. In but one, was it necessary to give anything special for the cough, and here an infusion of Red Clover answered the purpose well.

In the majority of cases of simple rubeola I prescribe: ℞ Tinct. Lobelia, (seed), gtts. x.; Tinct. Asclepias, gtts. xx. to xxx.; Water, ℥iv.; a teaspoonful every hour, Keep the patient quiet in bed, but not too warm. If need be, a sedative may be added to the medicine if the fever runs high.

CASE L.—*Rubeola—Tardy Appearance of the Eruption—Coma.*—S——, æt. ten years, has been exposed to measles, has the unpleasant appearance of the eyes, and the bronchial irritation so characteristic of the disease; is now the third day from attack. Skin dry and harsh, temperature high, pulse 140, has been unconscious for some six hours.

Prescribed—℞ Tinct. Aconite, gtts. v.; Tinct. Belladonna, gtts. x.; Water, ℥iv.; a teaspoonful every hour. The child gradually regained consciousness, though the eruption did not appear until the fifth day. After which small doses of Lobelia and Asclepias controlled the bronchial irritation.

CASE LI.—*Rubeola Maligna—Coma.*—Was called to see B——, æt. nine years, in a Fifth Street boarding house—all the surroundings bad. Is now in the seventh day of the disease, eruption has not made its appearance, has had two physicians who have given him up. Has not been conscious for three days.

Symptoms now: Pulse 120, oppressed, skin turgid and dusky red, face swollen, eyes reddened, breathes with difficulty from pulmonary congestion.

Ordered from the nearest drug store Acetous Emetic Tincture of the Dispensatory, and Compound Powder of Lobelia. Made an infusion of the last, and at once proceeded to administer them alternately, in small doses frequently repeated. In an hour, the stimulant influence was distinctly marked in an improved circulation and respiration. Thorough emesis in two hours, with speedy relief to the nervous system; and the patient was conscious, the eruption appearing freely in eight hours from first administration. Put the patient upon the use of: ℞ Tinct. Lobelia, gtts. x.; Tinct. Asclepias, gtts. xxx.; Water, ℥iv.; a teaspoonful every hour. Made a good recovery.

CASE LII.—*Rubeola Maligna.*—*Prof. Jones' Cases of Black Measles.*—Two brothers by the name of Baird, from Mason, Tenn., attending the Spring course of 1871, became sick, and after treating themselves for three or four days, sent for me. They were boarding themselves, and being alone in the room, had no attention.

Found the eldest brother sitting in his shirt and drawers, in a cold room, trying to build a fire, his face presenting that peculiar dark mottled appearance we observe after recovery from smallpox. Examination determined that it was measles, and a very unpleasant condition. Both cases were nearly alike—pulse 130 to 140, small and oppressed, eruption dusky, tongue *dark red*, dry, and covered with a brownish fur, sordes on teeth, cough very bad and expectorating largely a muco-pus—to the amount of a pint or more in twenty-four hours.

Prescribed—℞ Dilute Muriatic Acid, ℥j.; Simple Sirup, ℥ij.; add to water to make a pleasant drink and give freely. ℞ Tinct. Aconite, gtts. x.; Tinct. Asclepias, ℥ss.; Water, ℥iv.; a teaspoonful every hour. One showing a marked oppression of the nerve centres, and tendency to congestion, had Belladonna in place of the Asclepias for two days.

Their fellow students were very kind as soon as their situation became known, and kept the room of uniform temperature, and saw that they had food. We gave boiled milk and beef tea freely. Both convalesced well, and have had no subsequent trouble.

CASE LIII.—*Rubeola Maligna.*—M——, æt. 23, has had a chill, followed by high fever, a harsh dry cough, suffusion of eyes, with fullness and redness of skin. Now, the third day, the eruption shows itself, but does not come out freely.

Prescribed—Tinct. Aconite, gtts. x.; Tinct. Ipecac, gtts. xxx.; Water, ʒiv.; a teaspoonful every hour. A hot foot-bath and a cup of hot sage tea.

Saw him the next day—worse. The surface is somewhat dusky, eruption scant, tongue excessively dry. Prescribed in addition :℞ Sulphurous Acid, ʒj.; Simple Syrup, ʒij.; a teaspoonful every three hours. The unpleasant symptoms faded away rapidly, the eruption appeared, and the patient convalesced well.

CASE LIV.—*The Cough of Measles.*—A child of my own had measles during one of the severest endemics we ever had in this city, and as a sequel, had that persistent irritation of bronchii with cough, which is so unpleasant and so frequently fatal.

After an ineffectual use of the ordinary means, put her upon the use of: ℞ Tinct. Drosera, ʒss.; Water, ʒiv.; a teaspoonful four times a day. Was entirely relieved in a week or ten days, and though the cough would return with every slight cold, for a year following, it was always speedily checked by the same remedy. I have used the Drosera in scores of cases with like results, and now never think of prescribing anything but this or an infusion of Clover Hay.

Rheumatism.

The reader will notice that I do not propose to prescribe for the *name* rheumatism, any more than I would prescribe for the *name* "bilious fever." The cases of rheumatism only agree in one thing—the character of the pain ; and as we have long since learned, pain is only a symptom, and never to be prescribed for as *the* disease.

The reader may suggest, however, that writers agree that rheumatism is dependent upon the generation of lactic acid in excess, and that the deposit of this in the tissues is the cause of the local inflammation. And if so, surely the alkaline treatment so generally recommended, must be *the* treatment.

Whilst I admit the probability—that some product of retrograde metamorphosis, either of food or tissue, is the *materies morbi* in this disease, I am very sure it is not lactic acid ; and you will readily come to this conclusion if you will carefully read your Carpenter, Huxley or Draper. And I am quite as sure that there is in some an excess of alkalinity, in others an excess of acid, and in still others neither the one nor the other.

Case LV.—*Inflammatory Rheumatism.*—A. S., æt. 46, rheumatic diathesis, will have averaged an attack a year, for five years, running the usual course in about six weeks. Was called to attend him the third day of this attack—symptoms as follows :

Tongue clean, mucous membranes of normal color ; bowels regular ; pulse 110, full and oppressed ; some difficulty in respiration, and oppression in præcordia, requires to be propped up in bed ; the disease is localized in right knee, which is very much swollen, very painful, and exquisitely tender to the touch ; the most prominent symptom, as well as the most singular one, is the constant profuse sweating.

Prescribed—℞ Tinct. Aconite, gtts. xx.; Tinct. Macrotys, ℥ss.; Syrup, ℥ijss.; a teaspoonful every two hours—no effect only a severe headache. The next day he was put upon the use of alkalies, giving them freely in the form of Bicarbonate of Soda and Acetate of Potash — patient growing worse. With two days of this treatment changed to lemon juice, and gave Veratrum as the sedative—amendment for one day, and then a relapse. Sixth day of treatment gave Colchicum— English Wine, gtts. v. every two hours. Seventh day patient much worse. Colchicum has acted upon the bowels freely, and his stomach is irritable; sweating stopped whilst bowels were acting, but is now worse than ever. Eighth and ninth days a placebo; patient is suffering intensely, and talks of changing doctors. All this time we have been assiduous in making applications to the inflamed part, changing them from day to day, so that we have run through the entire list.

Reading up the treatment of phthisis a few weeks since I noticed the recommendation of a diaphoretic for night-sweats—have tried it in one case with advantage—why not give a diaphoretic for this prodigious sweating. And so I order that the patient be put between blankets, thoroughly rubbed down with dry flannel whenever the skin becomes wet, and give a strong infusion of Asclepias in tablespoonful doses. There was a decided amendment the first day, and by the fifteenth day of the disease the patient was convalescent.

CASE LVI.—*Inflammatory Rheumatism.*—George C., æt. 15, rheumatic diathesis, has had three very severe previous attacks, the last confining him to his bed ten weeks, and leaving serious structural heart disease—treatment Eclectic.

Symptoms as follows:—Now the third day; high fever; pulse 110, full and bounding; skin dry as parchment; urine scant and high-colored; bowels constipated; no appetite; mouth dry; mucous membranes natural as to color; tongue showing a clear white coat; is suffering intensely in one knee and ankle, the parts swollen, exquisitely tender and presenting evidences of active inflammation.

Prescribed—R Tinct. Veratrum, gtts. xx.; Tinct. Macrotys, gtts. xxx.; Water, ℥iv.; a teaspoonful every hour. Acetate
30

of Potash added to his drink in small quantity. Put the
patient between blankets, wrap the inflamed parts in flannel
and let them alone.

There was a gradual amendment, and the patient was convalescent by the ninth day, though the parts were weak, and
he did not get out of the house until the third week. But
what was most singular, the old heart disease was so improved, that he was comparatively free from suffering in this
respect, and the improvement continuing for some months,
even the marked saw-sound faded out, and to-day his heart
does its work well, with scarce a trace of disease.

CASE LVII.—*Inflammatory Rheumatism.*—Joseph B., æt.
41, is now in the second week of an attack of rheumatism,
the disease growing worse from day to day. Has had a Colchicum treatment with Mercury, with the common applications to the affected part.

Symptoms are all severe, but the one most pronounced, and
which indicates the line of treatment is—marked pallidity of
mucous membranes, broad pallid tongue, pitting where it
comes in contact with the teeth, and covered with a white
pasty coat.

Prescribed—Bicarbonate of Soda added to water, and give
freely as a drink. Inflamed parts to be wrapped in raw
cotton. Marked amendment in twenty-four hours, and
patient rapidly convalesced. No other remedy was given.

CASE LVIII.—*Inflammatory Rheumatism.*—K., æt. 30,
rheumatic diathesis, has lain for six or eight weeks in these
attacks ; presents the usual symptoms, disease located in lum-
bar region extending to hip.

Prescribed—℞ Tinct. Aconite,. gtts. x.; Tinct. Macrotys,
ℨss.; Water, ℨiv.; a teaspoonful every hour. Tongue shows
a slight increase of redness ; for which give lemonade. Fever
abates, and by the third day patient is apparently comfortable. Going on to the sixth day, there is a relapse, worse
than at first.

Notice a peculiar puffiness of hands and face, skin glistening, and for this give in addition to Aconite and Macrotys: R Acetate of Potash, ℥ss.; Tinct. Apocynum, gtts. xx.; Water, ℥ij.; a teaspoonful every three hours. Improves slowly, and the third day from this, drop the Acetate of Potash and give him Apocynum and Macrotys. Made a good recovery by the end of the week.

CASE LIX.—*Inflammatory Rheumatism.*—J. R. has been suffering from inflammatory rheumatism for more than three weeks; one of the worst cases I ever saw. Have treated him myself, and been assiduous in attention, using all the remedies recommended in such cases. Medicine has invariably made him worse, feels more comfortable when nothing is taken.

It is many years since, and just at that time Lemon Juice was recommended for rheumatism. Concluded to try it, but without any faith in its virtues, and gave it as freely as the patient could take it. There was amendment from the first, and before the end of the week he was very comfortable, and made a good recovery.

You ask me what was the indication for the Acid? I answer, that I don't know. I was treating names at that time, and my patient had "rheumatism."

I have not had a case of rheumatism in the past four years, in which the indications for an acid treatment were so marked, that I would have selected an acid alone; but I am sure I have had them in the earlier years of my practice.

CASE LX.—*Sub-Acute Rheumatism.*—M., æt. 35, of rheumatic diathesis, has been suffering since early Winter with sub-acute rheumatism. It shifts its position, and has affected most of the small articulations. There is slight œdema of the feet, and general puffiness of the skin, which presents a peculiar glistening appearance.

Prescribed—R Tinct. Apocynum Can., gtts. xx.; Water, ℥iv.; a teaspoonful every two hours. Improved steadily from the first, and the second week added Tinct. Nux Vomica, gtts. x.; taking the medicine every three hours. Was entirely free from the disease the third week.

CASE LXI.—*Sub-Acute Rheumatism.*—Chas. O. is suffering from a recent attack of sub-acute rheumatism. Two weeks since he applied for treatment for pain in the chest—costal rheumatism. Now it is located in the wrist and one phalangeal articulation.

Prescribed—R Tinct. Aconite, gtts. x.; Tinct. Macrotys, gtts. xx.; Water, ℥iv.; a teaspoonful every hour. The pain in the chest was removed with four doses of medicine, but the last attack required three days treatment.

I will not attempt to illustrate the treatment of chronic rheumatism, because it would be occupying space without advantage to the reader. It is especially difficult to describe a case of chronic disease, occupying some weeks of time, so that the reader can see the relation between symptoms and remedies.

In adddition to what has been pointed out, I may say, that we especially study the function of digestion and blood-making, and retrograde metamorphosis and excretion, for in some lesion of one of them we will probably find the disease constantly reproducing itself.

See that the act of digestion is properly performed, and that no morbid product is introduced into the circulation from the digestive apparatus. Then see that the waste of tissue goes on in a normal manner, and that all its products are removed as speedily as possible.

Infantile Pneumonia.

CASE LXII.—*Infantile Pneumonia.*—L., æt. four years, has been sick four days. The first day seemed to have a bad cold, the second had a chill, followed for two or three hours by fever. The third had a chill, followed by fever, which has continued up to the present in a remittent form. Both lungs are involved to a considerable extent, and the cough is harassing, sputa slightly "rusty." Pulse *full* and *open.*

Prescribed—℞ Tinct. Veratrum, gtts. x.; Water, ℥iv.; a teaspoonful every hour until the fever abates, then in half-teaspoonful doses. Apply to the chest a cloth spread with lard, and sprinkled with Comp. Powder of Lobelia. Convalescent with four days of treatment, the inflammatory action being arrested the first twenty-four hours.

CASE LXIII.—*Lobular Pneumonia, with Asthenic Bronchitis.*—N., æt. six months, has been sick for a week, gradually growing worse. Has a rattling cough, difficult respiration, remittent fever. Now seems very much prostrated, pulse small and frequent, no hardness; when the fever is on the child is very restless, when it goes off it seems exhausted. Mucus accumulates, and makes the breathing very difficu't.

Prescribed—℞ Tincture Lobelia, ℨj.; Compound Tincture of Lavender, ℨiij.; Simple Syrup, ℥jss. M. Give in small doses (¼ teaspoonful) every few minutes at first, then at intervals of an hour. The same local application to the chest as above.

In this case I gave the old formula. Now I very frequently add the Tincture of Lobelia Seed to water, and give it in the same manner as Veratrum and Aconite.

CASE LXIV.—*Infantile Pneumonia.*—G., æt. three years, has been sick but two days, yet looks to have been sick a week. Skin very dry and harsh, hot; pulse 130, small and sharp; tongue contracted and dry; a very persistent, dry, hacking cough; crepitation over a greater part of both lungs.

Prescribed—℞ Tinct. Aconite, gtts. viij.; Tinct. Ipecac,

ʒss.; Water, ℥iv.; a teaspoonful every hour. The plaster of
Lard with Emetic powder to the chest. Was *very* sick for
two days—breathing difficult. Amendment commenced the
third, and the child was convalescent by the sixth. No other
remedies were given.

This is a very common plan of treatment with me in these
cases, and it is rare to find one that does not yield readily.

CASE LXV. — *Infantile Pneumonia, with Congestion.*—S.,
æt. four years, has been sick twenty-four hours. Disease
commenced with a well marked chill, fever of an asthenic
character following. The child is semi-comatose, sleeps with
the eyes part open, eyes dull and pupils dilated; the toes are
cold; pulse 120, soft and easily compressed; cough in paroxysms, rattling, but no expectoration; an unpleasant rattling,
blowing sound heard over the larger portion of the chest—
the posterior part of the lung on right side is free. Had a
chill the second day, and again the third day.

Prescribed—℞ Tinct. Aconite, gtts. x.; Tinct. Belladonna,
gtts. x.; Water, ℥iv.; a teaspoonful every hour. Quinia inunction—℞ Quinia Sul., ʒj.; Adeps, ℥ij.; Oleum Anisi, gtts.
xx. M.—twice daily—to be throughly used. Emetic powder
and lard to chest.

The comatose symptoms were removed the first twelve
hours, the chill of the third day was lighter, and the child
was convalescent by the fifth day.

CASE LXVI.—*Infantile Pneumonia, with Determination to
the Brain.*—A., æt. twenty months, seemed to have had a bad
cold for a couple of days, the third day a very high fever
came up suddenly, the child being extremely restless, and had
a convulsion. Was called at this time. Found the skin hot—
not dry, pulse 140, sharp, mouth not dry but very red, eyes
bright, intolerant to light, pupils contracted to a point. A
very harassing hacking cough, respiration somewhat labored
and abdominal, small blowing sounds when the ear was applied to the chest.

Prescribed—℞ Tinct. Veratrum, gtts. x.; Tinct. Gelseminum, gtts. xxx.; Water, ℨiv.; a teaspoonful every hour. Same local application to the chest as before.

The unpleasant symptoms gradually yielded, and the child was convalescent on the fourth day of treatment.

I think these cases will illustrate pretty well the more frequent departures from the ordinary standard of infantile pneumonia, and the treatment necessary for the special forms of the disease. I have employed these remedies in this way for the ten years past—some of them for a longer time—and as they have not failed me when I have done my part to make a correct diagnosis, I recommend them to others with great confidence.

Cholera Infantum.

CASE LXVII.—*Cholera Infantum.*—M., æt. twenty-two months, is suffering from acute cholera infantum of three days' duration. Evacuations frequent, greenish, and attended with some tenesmus. Nausea with occasional vomiting; not as much thirst as is usual in the disease. A rare symptom in this disease, the pulse is *very full and strong*, ranging from 100 to 110 beats per minute.

I take the condition of the pulse as the key-note of the treatment, and prescribe—℞ Tincture Veratrum, gtts. x.; Water, ℨiv.; given in teaspoonful doses every hour until the fever declines and the patient is better, then half-teaspoonful doses.

No other remedy was given. There were but two discharges the third day; the fever had entirely disappeared. Ordered Quinine inunction once daily, and up to this time, the fourth week, there has been no return of the disease.

CASE LXVIII.—*Cholera Infantum.*—C., æt. twenty-eight months, has had diarrhœa since April, been treated by two physicians, always worse when taking medicine.

Skin sallow, relaxed and doughy; extremities cold, pulse soft, and easily compressed; tongue pale and covered with a dirty yellowish fur in streaks; vomits a yellow, unpleasant fluid mixed with mucus; discharges from the bowels mucoid, with a trace of pus and broken down blood.

Prescribed—℞ Triturated Podophyllin, 1-100th, one grain every two hours. Quinine inunction twice a day. A milk diet, care being used that the milk be sweet and good, and to which is added about ten grains of Phosphate of Soda in the twenty-four hours.

The child made a good recovery in two weeks, the amendment dating from the second day of treatment. I say the child made a recovery—for it is now eating well, gaining flesh, is walking, and plays with spirit, yet there is no doubt but it will have occasional slight attacks until cold weather.

CASE LXIX.—*Cholera Infantum.*—S., æt. two years, has had diarrhœa, thirst, and nausea and vomiting for three weeks, gradually increasing. Has taken Neutralizing Cordial, Bismuth, Ipecac, Hydrarg. Cum Creta, and astringents, without any good results—or rather with bad results, for the medicine has increased the disease.

Find on examination that the bowels are tumid, especially in hypochondria; there is umbilical pain at times, the skin is sallow and relaxed, the face especially is a sallow yellow, the tongue full, pale, and slightly dirty.

Prescribed—℞ Tinct. Nux Vomica, gtts. iij.; Water, ℥iv.; a teaspoonful every hour at first, then every two and three hours. The child made a good recovery in a week, no other remedy being given.

CASE LXX.—*Cholera Infantum.*—F., æt. twenty months, has had cholera infantum some nine weeks, is very much reduced, and the attending physician thinks recovery impossible. The evacuations from the bowels are copious and watery, some six or eight in the twenty-four hours; there is occasional nausea, such as would be produced by tickling the fauces, and the milk is almost uniformly thrown up after nursing.

There is one special feature—the child is dull and somnolent, the eyes dull and the pupils somewhat dilated and immobile.

The pulse is soft and easily compressed, the abdomen tumid with evident congestion of the portal circle.

Prescribed—℞ Tinct. Aconite, gtts. iv.; Tinct. Belladonna, gtts. x.; Water, ℥iv.; a teaspoonful every two hours. Amendment was perceptible the next day; the remedy was continued the first week, and then changed for small doses of Ipecac. The child made a good recovery.

These six cases will illustrate the specific treatment of cholera infantum or summer complaint. In ninety-five out of one hundred cases, the treatment will require but the three remedies, Ipecac, Aconite and Nux Vomica, one or more, but there are a few cases that require other means, and when specially indicated, we find they not only relieve the special symptoms, but the disease in its totality.

Dysentery.

CASE LXXI.—*Dysentery.*—G., æt. eight months, had diarrhœa, commencing in the morning, but in the evening the stools became small and bloody, attended with pain and tenesmus. Pulse 130 and hard, surface hot, very restless, nausea with occasional retching. Discharges about every ten minutes. Child regarded by the parents as in a dangerous condition, one having died in the same house from the same disease the week before.

Prescribed at 11 P. M.—℞ Tinct. Aconite, gtts. v.; Tinct. Ipecac, gtts. xv.; Water, ℥iv.; a teaspoonful every hour. No dysenteric discharges after 4 A. M. the next morning, and the child was well the second day.

CASE LXXII. — *Enteritis with Aphtha.* — Mary N., æt. seven months, was taken to church to be baptized during the cold spell the first of June. The child was considerably exposed, and the rector used water rather freely; the result a

31

severe cold with diarrhœa, and the third day a severe aphthous sore mouth.

Fever is constant—pulse ranging from 120 to 150 as the fever rises and falls: skin dry and harsh; discharges from the bowels profuse, greenish, and attended with pain; mouth hot and red; tongue red and partially coated; papillæ red and elongated; aphthous patches well defined and a clear pearly-white. Altogether the patient is very sick, and in the olden time the prognosis would have been very unfavorable.

Explained to the mother the character of the diarrhœa—that it was caused by inflammation of the small intestine, and that hence it would not do to check it suddenly—and that the sore mouth was but a symptom of the intestinal disease.

Prescribed—Tinct. Aconite, gtts. iij.; Tinct. Ipecac, gtts. v.; Water, ℥ij, (to be kept on ice); half a teaspoonful every half hour. Also, ℞ Tinct. Nux Vomica gtts. j.; Water, ℥ij.; to be given in teaspoonful doses as often as necessary to relieve the pain.

Slight amendment the second day, the discharges the same, but the fever not so high, and the pain controlled by the Nux. Not much change the third day, except that the aphthæ was slowly disappearing—difficulty thus far in persuading the friends that mouth washes were unnecessary. Added to the treatment Quinine inunction twice daily. The diarrhœa still continues the fourth day, but there is no pain or tenesmus, the fever has disappeared, the sore mouth is nearly gone, and the child is commencing to take milk and digest it.

Thus the case progressed with gradual amendment until the discharges became natural about the tenth day, and the child had a *perfect* recovery. But the father could not see why the diarrhœa should not be arrested at once, and was extremely anxious that large doses of some of the older remedies should be tried. Afterwards he expressed satisfaction that his solicitations were refused.

INDEX.

Tongue 276 (289), 252, 39, 47, 16, (384

32